Muscle Function Testing

Muscle Function Testing

Vladimír Janda   Professor of Neurology, Charles University, Prague
Head Physician, Rehabilitation Clinic, University Hospital,
Prague
Chief, Department of Rehabilitation Medicine, Postgraduate
Institute, Prague

Butterworths   London   Boston   Durban   Singapore   Sydney   Toronto
Wellington

English edition first published 1983

British Library Cataloguing in Publication Data

Janda, Vladimír
  Muscle function testing.
  1. Muscles—Motility
  I. Title   II. Vyšetřování hybnosti. *English*
  612'.74   QP321

ISBN 0-407-00201-4

Library of Congress Cataloging in Publication Data

Janda, Vladimír, Doc. MUDr.
  Muscle function testing.

  Bibliography: p.
  1. Muscles—Diseases—Diagnosis. 2. Joints—Range
of motion. 3. Function tests (Medicine) I. Title.
[DNLM: 1. Muscles—Physiology. 2. Muscular diseases—
Diagnosis. WE 500 J33v]
RC925.7.J35   1983   616.7'4075   83-7409
ISBN 0-407-00201-4

Phototypeset by Butterworths Litho Preparation Department
Printed and bound by Robert Hartnoll Ltd, Bodmin, Cornwall

Preface to the English edition

This book appeared first as a simple technical guide in the Czech language in 1979. Since that time, I have tried to re-evaluate different known tests, to refine them and eventually to add some new tests in the hope of providing more and better information for those working in this field. I was especially concerned to highlight the possible errors and mistakes which might occur during testing and which might thus decrease the validity of the assessment. It was my intention to present the instructions in such a form that any physiotherapist could undertake the tests without being guided and taught by another experienced person. One of the reasons for such an attempt lay in the fact that interest in detailed analysis of muscle function has decreased during the last several years. However, the recognition of the importance of the muscular system in various non-paralytic disorders of the osteoarticular system, as in back pain, and the demand for a better and more rational approach to therapeutic exercise led to the favourable reconsideration of methods which have been underestimated recently. Therefore this book was written as a practical manual for daily use.

It is my pleasant duty to thank all who helped in the preparation of this English edition. Among others, I would like to express my utmost thanks to Mrs Anne Signol for her stimulation and support and to Professor Margaret Bullock for the final revision of the manuscript. In was, indeed, not easy to prepare the English version from the Swedish translation. Last, but not least, my thanks are offered to Butterworths for the interest, effort and patience which they have shown to my book.

Vladimír Janda

Contents

Introduction

Muscle function testing is a method of examination that gives information about the following:

1. The strength of individual muscles or of muscle groups that form a functional unit.
2. The size, extent and progress of peripheral nerve lesions.
3. The nature of the simple movement patterns.
4. The conditions for analytical physiotherapy and determination of the work capacity of the part of the body being tested.

The tests are based on the fact that some muscle strength is always required to move a specific part of the body. This strength is adapted to the circumstances under which movement is carried out. In principle, muscle strength is graded as follows:

1. The muscle can overcome a resistance directed against the movement.
2. The muscle can overcome gravity.
3. The muscle can work, but only when gravity is eliminated.
4. The muscle can contract, but no movement results.

Muscle function testing is an analytical means of determining the strength of individual muscle groups. In recent years, opinions regarding the control of muscles have changed. The performance of movement is assessed to a far more complex degree and therefore muscle function testing now has greater importance.

At present muscle function testing has been reintroduced in a different form. Not only is the simple strength of an individual muscle or a synergistic muscle group tested, but in addition the whole movement pattern is assessed. The influence of neurological or reflex therapeutic methods has brought awareness that each movement depends on the coordination of several muscle groups often situated at a considerable distance from each other. It would be an oversimplification to say that muscle function testing involves simply the examination of an individual muscle of one muscle group. Modern muscle function testing examines certain very carefully defined, standardized and relatively simple movement patterns.

In other words, muscle function testing is no longer limited to the measurement of muscle strength and includes observations of the performance of the movement and the sequence of activation of the individual muscle groups that are principally involved. It is not restricted to peripheral motor lesions since inhibition of muscles and changed movement patterns and habits are also taken into account. Consequently the technique of distinguishing small variations within the normal range has become more and more important. Special tests to estimate movement patterns have had to be evolved.

The development of these testing methods can be traced back to the period before the First World War when R W Lovett used a manual approach for the first time to assess muscle strength in children with poliomyelitis. The examination technique has become more accurate but the principle is the same. In 1946 the method was re-evaluated by the National Foundation for Infantile Paralysis in the USA. In 1947 Daniels, Williams and Worthingham published a book in which the procedure was discussed in detail. As far as can be determined from a survey of the literature, the essential features of muscle function testing remain unchanged. The techniques in this book are based on the same principles. However, particular tests have been modified, refined or completely changed and others newly introduced.

Attempts to measure muscle strength and also indirectly motion in general have been made for a long time. Many have not been successful because of simple disadvantages. Although a number of ergometers and machines with measurable resistance have been employed, the majority are not suitable for practical use because they are difficult to handle and not all muscles can be tested with them. Graphical methods have gained more importance in recent years, and among these electromyography is pre-eminent so far as assessment of the locomotor system is concerned. Manual muscle tests have undoubted disadvantages – for example they only show the momentary state of the muscle – but with a basic knowledge of anatomy, physiology and kinesiology it is not difficult to understand their principles and applications. To avoid as far as possible the risk of introducing error it is important to keep to the prescribed procedures and to avoid individual modifications.

The method of grading muscle strength has changed several times, although the principles have remained the same. While different authors use their own systems the simplified 1946 classification is most common. This method divides muscle strength into six groups as follows:

Grade 5: N (normal). A normal, very strong muscle with a full range of movement and able to overcome considerable resistance. This does not mean that the muscle is normal in all circumstances (for example, when at the onset of fatigue or in a state of exhaustion).

Grade 4: G (good). A muscle with good strength and a full range of movement, and able to overcome moderate resistance.

Grade 3: F (fair). A muscle with a complete range of movement against gravity only when resistance is not applied.

Grade 2: P (poor). A very weak muscle with a complete range of motion only when gravity is eliminated by careful positioning of the patient.

Grade 1: T (trace). A muscle with evidence of slight contractility but no effective movement.

Grade 0: A muscle with no evidence of contractility.

The grades are designated by arabic numbers. Percentages are not used because they are not an appropriate way of recording muscle strength. If the strength of the muscle lies between two grades, a plus or minus sign can be used.

Testing of facial muscles is often neglected, and so in this book a grading system has been introduced for them. The muscle strength is calculated by comparing the movements of the paralysed and the normal sides. Six grades are used. To achieve better muscle relaxation the subject is tested in supine lying which is important especially for grades 0−2. Facial muscle strength is graded as follows:

Grade 5: Normal muscle contraction and no asymmetry compared with the normal side.

Grade 4: Almost normal contraction and very little asymmetry compared with the normal side.

Grade 3: Muscle contraction on the paralysed side gives about half the normal range of movement.

Grade 2: Muscle contraction on the paralysed side produces a quarter of the normal range of movement.

Grade 1: When movement is attempted there is evident muscle contraction.

Grade 0: When movement is attempted there is no muscle contraction.

To perform a muscle function test properly it is essential to have a detailed knowledge of individual muscles and their movements. Careful assessment is impossible or very difficult in certain circumstances, above all when there is a decreased range of movement, substitution, incoordination (see page 5) or pain. It must be stressed that muscle function testing is not suitable in cases of spastic paralysis or progressive muscular dystrophy. Performance of the test is made more difficult, or even impossible, if the range of movement is limited by anatomical changes in the joint, pain, changes in the connective tissues, contractures, and so on. In order to achieve maximal standardization and simplification the best position for the activation of some muscles cannot be utilized.

With respect to a certain movement the muscles have the following relationships:

1. Prime movers (agonists) take the greatest part in the movement.
2. Assisting muscles (synergists) do not carry out the movement but help the prime mover and may partly compensate if it is paralysed.
3. Antagonists perform motion in the opposite direction. These muscles are passively stretched during the movement and in normal circumstances this does not influence its range. However, if they are shortened they may substantially limit the movement.
4. Stabilizers do not perform the movement but fix the relevant part of the body in a constant position so that motion can

take place in the right direction. Poor fixation sometimes results in a decrease of the final strength. During assessment, therefore, fixation is of great importance. If possible, external fixation is supplied by the examiner's hand so that the action of the stabilizers is eliminated or diminished. As a rule, when testing a two-joint muscle good fixation is essential. The same applies to all muscles in children and in adults whose cooperation is poor and whose movements are incoordinated and weak. The better the extremity is steadied, the less the stabilizers are activated and the better and more accurate are the results of the muscle function test. When fixation is inadequate the prime mover cannot work fully. At a later check of the test the function of the stabilizers may have improved so that they work better. The movement is more exact and the final result is better, and the prime mover is assessed incorrectly.

5. Neutralizers abolish the second component of the normal direction of movement due to the prime mover. Each muscle functions in at least two directions corresponding to its anatomical position. If it is a flexor and a supinator then for pure flexion a muscle group with a pronator function must be activated and the supinator component neutralized. A muscle can at the same time be a synergist and a neutralizer. For example, in flexion of the elbow the prime mover is the biceps and its action has a component of supination. The pronator teres pronates the lower arm and is also a weak flexor of the elbow. If flexion alone is required, the flexor components of both muscles are added and the rotator components neutralized. Neutralizers are of great importance in daily life, but in muscle function testing they are a nuisance. Their action is greatly diminished by correct positioning of the extremities to allow accurate resistance and good fixation.

Range of movements

One of the most important principles of muscle function testing is that the movement must be performed to its greatest possible extent. There are several causes of decreased movement and the most important are the following:

1. Weakness of the prime mover so that it cannot perform the full range of movement.
2. Antagonists that are contracted or shortened so that the agonist cannot carry out the movement.
3. Anatomical changes in the joint so that the full movement cannot be performed.
4. Pain limiting the range of motion.

These principal points should be investigated before testing commences. The joints must be moved passively beforehand, and if the patient complains of pain then the movement must not be forced actively or passively to the limit. Findings are recorded using the following abbreviations: LR (limited range, with a short description of cause); C (contracture); SC (strong contracture); S (spasm); and SS (strong spasm). There should also be a description of the respective muscle or tissue.

Substitution and incoordination

The meanings of the terms substitution and incoordination have changed considerably, especially as a result of the influence of facilitation and reflex techniques. At first substitution is not, as a rule, recommended because there is a risk that the patient will develop undesirable movement patterns which can be changed later only with great difficulty. Although substitution can be

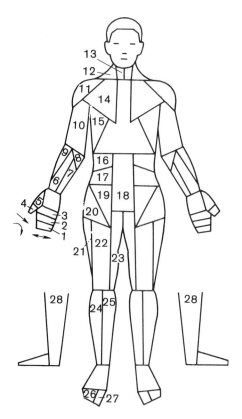

Diagram of muscle groups
⟷ mm. interossei palmares, → m. adductor pollicis⌢m. opponens pollicis, (1) m. flexor digitorum profundus, (2) m. flexor digitorum superficialis, (3) mm. lumbricales, (4) m. flexor pollicis longus, (5) m. flexor pollicis brevis, (6) m. flexor carpi radialis, (7) m. flexor carpi ulnaris, (8) m. pronator teres, (9) m. brachioradialis, (10) m. biceps brachii, (11) m. deltoideus, (12) m. trapezius, (13) m. sternocleidomastoideus, (14) m. pectoralis, (15) m. serratus anterior, (16) mm. obliqui externi abdominis, (17) m. transversus, (18) m. rectus abdominis, (19) m. iliopsoas, (20) m. sartorius, (21) m. tensor fasciae latae, (22) m. quadriceps femoris, (23) mm. adductores, (24) m. tibialis anterior, (25) m. tibialis posterior, (26) m. extensor digitorum, (27) m. extensor hallucis, (28) mm. peronei

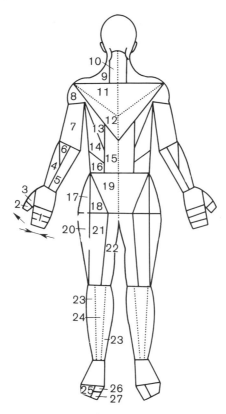

Diagram of muscle groups
→ ← mm. interossei dorsales, ← mm. abductores pollicis, (1) m. extensor digitorum, (2) m. extensor pollicis longus, (3) m. extensor pollicis brevis, (4) mm. extensores carpi radialis, (5) m. extensor carpi ulnaris, (6) m. supinator, (7) m. triceps brachii, (8) m. deltoideus, (9) m. trapezius (over fibrous tissue), (10) m. erector spinae, (11) m. trapezius (in middle and under fibrous tissue), (12) m. infraspinatus, (13) m. teres major, (14) m. latissimus dorsi, (15) m. erector spinae, (16) m. quadratus lumborum, (17) m. gluteus medius, (18) lateral rotators, (19) m. gluteus maximus, (20) m. tensor fasciae latae, (21) m. biceps femoris, (22) semitendinosus and m. semimembranosus, (23) m. gastrocnemius, (24) m. soleus, (25) mm. lumbricales, (26) m. flexor hallucis brevis, (27) m. flexor hallucis longus

useful, because it may compensate for absent function, this is not the case with incoordination. The cause of incoordination is difficult to ascertain and cannot be explained by the laws of biomechanics explained above. The old classification of incoordination is retained only for teaching purposes. The categories are as follows:

1. Incoordination of one muscle.
2. Incoordination of a synergistic muscle group.
3. Incoordination among antagonistic muscle groups.
4. Incoordination of muscle groups that bear no functional relationship.

Incoordination is regarded principally as a disturbance of motor regulation, either in the degree of activation or in the timing of individual groups. It appears within a certain movement pattern and leads among other things to an overstressed joint, decreased performance and premature exhaustion of the muscle.

Technical rules

To perform muscle function tests properly the following principles must be observed:

1. With a few exceptions, the whole range of movement and not only the beginning or end of the range must be tested.
2. Movement must take place at an even speed throughout.
3. Fixation must be as steady as possible.
4. At the point of fixation neither the tendon nor the muscle must be under pressure.
5. Resistance must be applied continuously and always against the direction of movement.
6. Resistance must be applied with uniform strength throughout.
7. Resistance must not be applied over two joints.
8. The patient must start to perform the movement as he is accustomed to. Only after recording the movement pattern is it corrected if necessary.

The assessment should take place in a warm room where every distraction has been eliminated. The examination plinth must be firm, sufficiently long and wide, with an even surface and without rounded edges. The examiner should have a friendly manner, especially if it is the patient's first visit. The examination should not be hurried because it can be accurate only if it is performed slowly. Beforehand, the examiner should explain the purpose of the assessment and emphasize that it is pain-free. During the tests individual movements should be explained to the patient in a concise fashion. Basic psychological principles apply not only in physiotherapy but also in the assessment itself, and patient cooperation can be obtained more readily just by talking in a relaxed manner. At the same time the practitioner gets better results and the tests proceed more quickly and pleasantly.

Muscle function tests should be repeated regularly, and by so doing their value is increased. It is desirable for the assessment to be performed by the same person each time. Repeated tests will show improvement or deterioration of the patient as well as revealing whether treatment is being properly carried out. Muscle function tests must be performed accurately, otherwise it is impossible to compare results from different examiners.

Observations and notes on the muscle function tests performed, including any discrepancies that are detected, must be recorded on proper forms. If by any chance the tests have not been carried out correctly, this must also be recorded. In such cases it is better to use the forms shown on pages 252–260, and to note the strengths of the different muscles.

Section 1 Muscle function testing: individual parts

Part 1 The face

The facial muscles are divided into three groups as follows:

1. The mimic muscles of facial expression innervated by the facial nerve (seventh cranial nerve). They are typical skin muscles without any deep fascia. At least one of their attachments invariably inserts into either the skin or the mucous membrane.
2. The muscles of mastication innervated by the trigeminal nerve (fifth cranial nerve). They comprise the masseter, temporalis, pterygoideus lateralis and pterygoideus medialis. These muscles protrude, retract, elevate, depress and move the mandible from side to side, and in addition adduct the jaws, that is close the mouth.
3. The ocular muscles, including the levator palpebrae superioris.

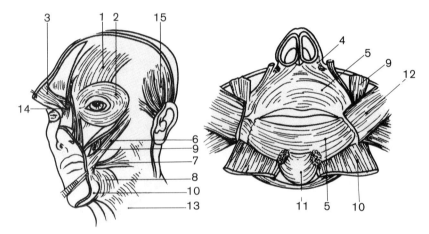

The facial muscles
(1) m. frontalis, (2) m. orbicularis oculi, (3) m. corrugator supercilii, (4) m. nasalis, (5) m. orbicularis oris, (6) m. zygomaticus major, (7) m. risorius, (8) m. depressor anguli oris, (9) m. levator anguli oris, (10) m. depressor labii interioris, (11) m. mentalis, (12) m. buccinator, (13) m. platysma, (14) m. procerus, (15) m. temporalis

The muscles of the tongue and the palate are not discussed here.
Movement of the mandible takes place at the temporomandibular joints. There is a marked difference between the joint surfaces and their junction is made smoother by an articular disc. The mechanism of movement in the temporomandibular joint is

very complex. The condyle of the mandible articulates with the undersurface of the articular disc in a hinge movement and the disc itself moves in a gliding action. Both gliding and hinge movements are equally involved in depression (that is, abduction and opening the mouth) and elevation (that is, adduction and closing the mouth) of the mandible. When the mandible is moved from side to side, as in grinding, protraction must be carried out on one side and simultaneous retraction on the other. The chin moves towards the retracted side.

The mimic muscles of facial expression

Frontalis

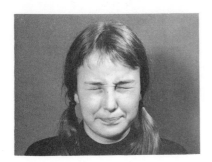

Origin: The anterior border of the galea aponeurotica.
Insertion: Blends with the skin and muscles of the forehead above the eyebrow and the glabella.
Action: Raises the eyebrow and the skin over the root of the nose. Wrinkles the forehead transversely and assists in opening the eye.

Orbicularis oculi

Origin: The medial palpebral ligament, the frontal process of the maxilla and the crest of the lacrimal bone.
Insertion: The central palpebral fibres lie within the eyelid and are attached by the medial palpebral ligament to the frontal process of the maxilla. The peripheral orbital fibres surround the orbital margin and are attached medially to the medial palpebral ligament and directly to the frontal process of the maxilla.
Action: This is the sphincter muscle of the eyelid. The palpebral part can act involuntarily to close the lid gently such as in sleep, winking and blinking. The orbital portion is voluntary and is used in frowning.

Corrugator supercilii

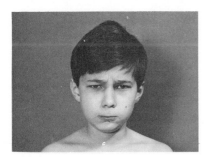

Origin: The medial end of the superciliary arch.
Insertion: Into the deep surface of the skin above the middle of the supraorbital margin.
Action: Draws the eyebrow medially and downwards forming vertical wrinkles.

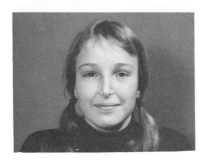

Nasalis

Origin: Above the upper front teeth from the maxilla just lateral to the nasal notch.
Insertion: Into the nasal cartilage and ala nasi.
Action: Compresses the nasal aperture.

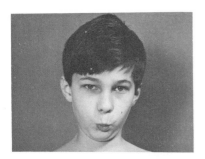

Orbicularis oris

This is the sphincter surrounding the mouth and it forms the greater part of the substance of the lips.
Action: Moves the lips to close the mouth in a pouting action and produces a small orifice such as in whistling.

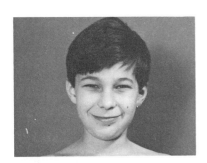

Zygomaticus major

Origin: The zygomatic bone in front of the zygomaticotemporal suture.
Insertion: Into the angle of the mouth.
Action: Draws the angle of the mouth upwards and laterally such as in laughing.

Risorius

Origin: The parotid fascia.
Insertion: Into the skin at the angle of the mouth.
Action: Retracts the angle of the mouth and forms dimples in the cheeks.

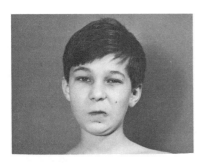

Levator anguli oris

Origin: Canine fossa.
Insertion: Into the skin at the angle of the mouth.
Action: Raises the angle of the mouth and assists in producing the nasolabial furrow and showing the teeth.

Depressor labii inferioris

Origin: The oblique line of the mandible.
Insertion: Into the skin of the lower lip and chin.
Action: Draws the lower lip downwards and a little laterally, such as in the expression of irony.

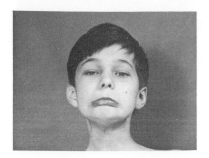

Depressor anguli oris

Origin: The oblique line of the mandible.
Insertion: Into the skin at the angle of the mouth.
Action: Draws the angle of the mouth downwards and laterally such as in the expression of sadness.

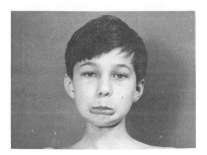

Mentalis

Origin: The incisive fossa of the mandible.
Insertion: Into the skin of the chin.
Action: Raises and protrudes the lower lip and at the same time wrinkles the skin of the chin, expressing doubt or disdain.

Buccinator

Origin: The outer surface of the alveolar processes of the maxilla and the mandible opposite the three molar teeth and, behind, the anterior border of the pterygomandibular raphe.
Insertion: Into the skin of the lips at the angle of the mouth.
Action: This muscle forms the majority of the substance of the cheek. It compresses the cheek against the teeth so that the food is kept between the teeth in chewing. When the cheek is distended with air, this muscle expels it between the lips in forced blowing. It also assists in widening the mouth such as in laughing and crying.

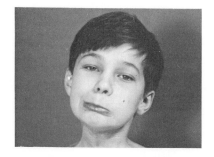

Platysma

Origin: The fascia covering the upper parts of the pectoralis major and the deltoid at the level of the second and third ribs.
Insertion: Some fibres are inserted into the lower border of the body of the mandible, some into the skin and subcutaneous tissue of the lower part of the face and many blend with the muscles around the angle and the lower part of the mouth.
Action: Assists in drawing down the lower lip and the angle of the mouth such as in the expression of horror or surprise. This muscle is a weak depressor of the jaw and it wrinkles the surface of the skin of the neck and tends to diminish the concavity between the jaw and the side of the neck. The external jugular vein lies under the platysma.

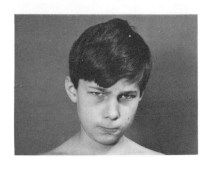

Procerus

Origin: The fascia covering the lower part of the nasal bone and the upper part of the lateral nasal cartilage.
Insertion: Into the skin over the lower part of the forehead between the eyebrows.
Action: Draws down the medial angle of the eyebrow and produces a transverse furrow over the bridge of the nose.

The muscles of mastication

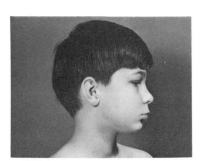

Masseter

Origin: The zygomatic arch.
Insertion: Into the lateral surface of the ramus and the angle of the mandible.
Action: Elevates the mandible and presses it against the maxilla such as in clenching the teeth.

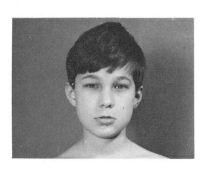

Temporalis

Origin: The temporal fossa.
Insertion: Into the coronoid process and the anterior border of the ramus of the mandible.
Action: Elevates and retracts the mandible.

Pterygoideus lateralis

Origin: By two heads from the lateral surface of the lateral pterygoid plate and the infratemporal surface of the greater wing of the sphenoid.
Insertion: Into a depression on the front of the neck of the mandible and into the articular capsule and disc of the temporomandibular joint.
Action: Protrudes and depresses the mandible and assists opening of the mouth.

Pterygoideus medialis

Origin: By two heads from the medial surface of the lateral pterygoid plate and the maxillary tuberosity.
Insertion: Into the medial surface of the ramus and the angle of the mandible.
Action: Elevates and protrudes the mandible.

Part 2 The trunk

The vertebral column forms the central axis of the skeleton. The trunk consists of the vertebral column with the ribs, the sternum and the pelvis. The column itself is composed of 34 vertebrae: seven cervical, 12 thoracic, five lumbar, five sacral and five coccygeal. All the vertebrae are united in two ways; first to their adjacent vertebrae, forming the "motion segment" of Junghanns, and secondly all together by the longitudinal ligaments common to all of them. Between the vertebral bodies are 24 intravertebral discs which are fibrocartilaginous and contribute about a quarter of the length of the column. The disc acts as a shock absorber and has a specific importance at each movement.

The vertebrae and the discs form a flexible pillar with distinct curvatures. Those in the sagittal plane are known as lordosis and kyphosis. Normal secondary curvatures of the vertebral column are cervical lordosis, thoracic kyphosis, lumbar lordosis and sacral and coccygeal kyphosis. Abnormal deviation in the lateral plane is known as scoliosis and is defined as left or right depending on the side of the convexity.

Movement of the vertebral column takes place between adjacent vertebrae. The range of movements is limited but they augment each other so that the final result is great flexibility. Motion is most marked in the cervical region, particularly at the atlanto-occipital and atlantoaxial joints. Motion is least marked in the thoracic region due to the rib joints. The basic movements of the vertebral column are flexion, extension, side-flexion, rotation and springy movements in the direction of the central axis which are connected with the normal curvature of the vertebral column. Flexion, extension and side-flexion are maximal in the cervical and lumbar regions.

The thorax is formed by 12 pairs of ribs which articulate posteriorly with the thoracic vertebrae and anteriorly with the sternum. Each rib consists of a bony posterior and lateral portion and a cartilaginous anterior portion. The upper seven ribs articulate through the costal cartilages with the sternum and are known as the true ribs, the eighth to 10th ribs articulate through the costal cartilages with the cartilage immediately above and are called false ribs, and the 11th and 12th ribs have free anterior ends and are known as floating ribs. The ribs are of different lengths such that the first is short and the consecutive ones increase in length until the seventh and thereafter become shorter. The sternum is a flat bone which articulates with the clavicles and the costal cartilages. A typical rib articulates posteriorly with the corresponding vertebrae in two places, but movement is only possible if it is simultaneous in both joints.

13

Because all the ribs articulate with each other and with the sternum there is no isolated movement of any one rib. On elevation of the ribs the volume of the thoracic cavity is increased and inspiration occurs.

Nerve supply

Innervation of the cervical region is supplied by the cervical plexus which is formed from the anterior primary rami of the upper four cervical nerves. These have both sensory and motor branches. The most important is the phrenic nerve which descends through the neck and the thorax to supply the diaphragm. Other branches to the muscles supply the prevertebral muscles, the scalenus and the vertebral muscles, and partly the sternocleidomastoideus and the trapezius. The last two also derive some nerve fibres from the spinal accessory nerve or the eleventh cranial nerve.

The thoracic nerves do not form a plexus and the segmental innervation is maintained. These nerves are mixed and supply both muscles and skin. The anterior primary rami of the thoracic spinal nerves form the intercostal nerves which run in the intercostal spaces to supply the intercostales, the transversus thoracis, the serratus posterior inferior, the serratus posterior superior and the abdominal muscles. The abdominal muscles are also served by the lumbar plexus. The posterior ramus of the thoracic nerves innervates the extensor muscles of the back before ending in medial and lateral cutaneous branches which supply the skin of the back. The nerve supply of the trunk is fairly simple.

Muscles

According to their relationship with the vertebral column the muscles of the trunk are divided into a dorsal group, that is muscles of the back and the back of the neck, and an anterior group, that is abdominal, neck, anterior chest wall and pelvic girdle muscles.

Dorsal group

The muscles of the back and the back of the neck comprise the following:

1. A superficial spinohumeral layer attaching the shoulder girdle to the trunk. These are flat muscles and belong to the upper extremity.
2. An intermediate spinocostal layer innervated by intercostal nerves.
   (a) Serratus posterior superior. This arises from the spines of the sixth cervical vertebra and the upper two or three

14

thoracic vertebrae and inserts by four digitations into the second to fifth ribs. It elevates the ribs and takes part in inspiration.

(b) Serratus posterior inferior. This arises from the spines of the lower two thoracic and upper two or three lumbar vertebrae, and inserts by four digitations into the lower four ribs. It depresses the ribs and takes part in expiration.

3. A deep layer. These are the true muscles of the back.

(a) Short muscles close to the vertebral column connecting contiguous vertebrae with each other. Their exact function has not been established.

(i) The interspinales are found between the spines of contiguous vertebrae. They tilt the vertebrae.

(ii) The intertransversarii. These also tilt the vertebrae.

(iii) The suboccipital muscles. These move in the junction between the vertebral column and the head. The rectus capitis posterior minor extends the head backwards on bilateral contraction and rotates the head on unilateral contraction. The rectus capitis posterior major acts as a synergist to the above muscle and in addition assists in rotation of the head. The obliquus capitis superior acts as a synergist to the two recti. (All these muscles are employed more frequently as postural muscles than as prime movers.) The obliquus capitis inferior turns the atlas vertebra, and hence the face, towards the same side.

(iv) The rotatores. These are eleven in number on each side in the thoracic region. Their action produces rotation.

(v) The coccygeus. This is triangular and passes from the spine of ischium to the sides of the lower sacrum and the coccyx.

(b) Long muscles connecting vertebrae that are not immediately adjacent to each other. This group consists of a vast muscle mass that is not completely differentiated and includes a large number of muscles in different layers. They all have similar actions. On unilateral contraction they produce lateral flexion and rotation of the vertebral column and on bilateral contraction they extend the vertebral column, hence the name erector spinae.

(i) Lateral column: iliocostalis lumborum, iliocostalis thoracis and iliocostalis cervicis.

(ii) Intermediate column: longissimus thoracis, longissimus cervicis and longissimus capitis.

(iii) Medial column: spinalis thoracis, spinalis cervicis and spinalis capitis.

(iv) Transversospinalis: this is a new term for previously differentiated muscles comprising the semispinales, multifidi and rotatores.

Anterior group

It is impossible to test the coccygeus and the muscles of the pelvic floor and they are not described further. The muscles of the head have been dealt with above.

15

The muscles of the neck are situated between the skull, the vertebral column and the thorax. The platysma, which is a muscle of facial expression, and the sternocleidomastoideus also belong here. The function of the sternocleidomastoideus and of the muscles above and below the hyoid bone is described in the section on testing. The scaleni are particularly important. They raise and fix the ribs and enable forced inspiration when the head is fixed. When the ribs are fixed they act as flexors of the head and the neck on bilateral contraction while on unilateral contraction they act as flexors to the same side and rotators to the opposite side. The longus capitis and longus colli lie on the anterior aspect of the vertebral column. On bilateral contraction they flex the head forwards and on unilateral contraction they flex it to the same side. The oblique muscle fibres of the longus colli take part in rotation of the vertebral column. The short intertraversarii anteriores cervicis and the rectus capitis lateralis lie on the lateral aspect of the vertebral column. They enable flexion of the vertebrae and the head towards the same side.

Muscles of the thoracic cage form the following groups:

1. The true muscles of the thoracic wall.
2. The muscles connecting the upper limb to the trunk (these are described together with the muscles of the upper limb).
3. The diaphragm with its specialized function.

The true muscles of the thoracic wall are very closely connected with the bony parts of the thorax. They lie between the ribs filling the intercostal spaces and they approximate the ribs in an elastic fashion. They participate mainly in respiration. These muscles are as follows:

1. The intercostales externi. These descend obliquely forwards from the lower border of the rib above to the upper border of the rib below (posterior and superior to anterior and inferior). They elevate the ribs and act as muscles of inspiration. Levatores costarum breves and longi are identical in function and development with the intercostales externi.
2. The intercostales interni. These descend obliquely backwards, depressing the ribs and taking part in expiration.
3. The transversus thoracis. This depresses the upper costal cartilages and assists in expiration, although it is of very small functional value.

The diaphragm is a muscular and tendinous septum separating the thoracic and abdominal cavities. It is convex towards the thoracic cavity. The peripheral muscular component can be divided into vertebral, costal and sternal parts according to origin. The central portion is tendinous. The diaphragm is the most important muscle of inspiration. During contraction the dome of the diaphragm descends and flattens so that the vertical diameter of the chest is increased, the intrathoracic pressure is decreased and the lungs expand to facilitate filling of the heart and to assist in venous return. The diaphragm and the abdominal muscles, which contract simultaneously, are responsible for the increase in the intra-abdominal pressure.

The most important muscles of inspiration are the intercostales externi, the diaphragm, the levatores costarum breves and the levatores costarum longi. The muscles assisting inspiration are the muscles of the anterior abdominal wall, the intercostales, the rhomboidei, the serratus anterior, the trapezius, the pectoralis major, the pectoralis minor, the latissimus dorsi and the subclavius.

The main muscles of expiration are the intercostales interni, the intercostales externi and the transversus thoracis. The muscles assisting expiration are the muscles of the anterior abdominal wall, the iliocostales, the longissimus thoracis, the serratus posterior inferior and the quadratus lumborum.

The muscles of the thoracic cage cannot be tested in the same way as the other skeletal muscles. Only through close observation of the breathing pattern can the participation of individual muscles be measured.

Muscles of the abdomen

The abdominal wall is formed by a group of five flat muscles which are connected anatomically and functionally. They are strengthened by many fasciae and aponeuroses.

The abdominal muscles have many different origins and insertions. Some attach not to the bone but to the ligaments or aponeuroses of other muscles. The abdominal muscles work as a unit and all participate in every movement of the trunk, although not always in the same relationship to each other. They act as muscles of expiration and during rest support the abdominal viscera and keep them under constant pressure. They also assist in expulsive efforts such as defaecation, micturition and vomiting. The abdominal muscles act in flexion, rotation and lateral flexion of the trunk. They contract maximally during all movements when the sternum approximates the symphysis pubis, that is when the thoracic and lumbar spine becomes kyphotic. The individual actions of the abdominal muscles, in particular rotation, have been questioned. The origin and insertion of these muscles are often separated by other tissue so that bundles of muscle fibres run separately. Some muscles are composed of many functional units.

The rectus abdominis is the vertical abdominal muscle. Its origins are the fifth, sixth and seventh costal cartilages and the xiphoid process. The fibres descend and insert on the pubic crest and on the front of the pubic symphysis. This muscle acts during lumbar and lower thoracic flexion, which is not the same as flexion of the whole trunk.

The obliquus externus abdominis is the outer diagonal abdominal muscle. It is the strongest of the diagonal muscles. It originates from the outer surfaces of the lower eight ribs and inserts onto the iliac crest, the xiphoid process, the linea alba and the front of the body of the pubis. The fibres run in an anterior inferior direction and the most inferior ones run almost completely vertically. The superior fibres originate from the fifth to the seventh costal cartilages and act in compression of the thorax and assist the initiation of flexion. The middle part has its origins in the seventh to ninth costal cartilages and is to a large extent an extension of the middle part of the obliquus internus abdominis. On unilateral contraction it acts as a rotator to the opposite side and on bilateral contraction it assists in flexion. The inferior part of the obliquus externus abdominis contains fibres that run from the last three ribs to the iliac crest. This is the only portion with both a bony origin and a bony insertion. These fibres run in a very diagonal fashion and act in side-flexion as well as rotation. On bilateral contraction they also assist in extension. When the pelvis is fixed the obliquus externus abdominis on unilateral contraction rotates the thorax to the opposite side, and on bilateral contraction depresses the ribs and assists in trunk flexion. It also contributes to side-flexion and extension.

The obliquus internus abdominis is the inner diagonal abdominal muscle. Its origins are the thoracolumbar fascia, the iliac crest and the inguinal ligament. The muscle fibres spread out like a fan. The superior fibres insert into the costal margin of the last three ribs and ascend superiorly and medially. Their function resembles that of the inferior part of the obliquus externus abdominis, that is on unilateral contraction they act to rotate the trunk to the same side and on bilateral contraction they assist in extension of the trunk. The middle fibres form an aponeurosis which splits around the upper part of the rectus abdominis and inserts into the linea alba. These fibres pass superiorly and medially. Their function corresponds to that of the same part of the obliquus externus abdominis, that is they assist in rotation and flexion. The inferior part of the obliquus internus abdominis contains fibres that pass anteriorly and medially and slightly inferiorly. They insert onto the pubis and into the linea alba and due to this do not take part in rotation or flexion, but only support the transversus abdominis during compression of the abdominal wall. To sum up, on unilateral contraction the obliquus internus abdominis assists in trunk rotation, turning the body to the same side. On bilateral contraction it assists slightly in trunk flexion. It is also activated during back extension.

The transversus abdominis is the horizontal abdominal muscle. It originates from the seventh to 12th costal cartilages, the thoracolumbar fascia, the anterior two thirds of the iliac crest and the lateral third of the inguinal ligament. It inserts into the aponeurosis of the obliquus internus abdominis. All the fibres run in a horizontal fashion and form a support for the abdominal contents. The transversus abdominis probably does not take part directly in the movements of the trunk, but provides a suitable background for the other muscles. When the muscle is weak a false hernia is created.

The quadratus lumborum has its origin at the inferior border of the 12th rib and inserts onto the transverse processes of the lower three or four lumbar vertebrae and into the iliolumbar ligament and the adjacent part of the iliac crest. It assists in side-flexion. When the thorax is fixed the quadratus lumborum elevates the pelvis on the same side and on bilateral contraction it assists in fixation of the vertebral column.

1 The neck:

Flexion

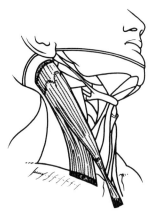

Position of the flexion muscle in the neck, m. sternocleidomastoideus

	C1	C2	C3	C4	C5	C6	C7	C8	Muscle
					C5	C6	C7		M. scalenus anterior (ventr.)
		C2	C3	C4	C5	C6	C7	C8	M. scalenus medius
						C6	C7	C8	M. scalenus posterior (dors.)
		C2	C3	C4	C5	C6	C7		M. longus colli
	C1	C2	C3						M. longus capitis
N. accessorius	C1	C2	C3						M. sternocleido-mastoideus

General comments

The basic movements are flexion of the neck by an arc-like movement of the head towards the sternum (forward flexion), flexion of the head by the head jutting forwards, and flexion of the neck together with rotation of the head.

Grades 5, 4, 3, 1 and 0 are tested in supine lying and grade 2 in side lying. Usually the right and left sides are examined at the same time. However, grades 5, 4 and 3 may be tested one side at a time, which is particularly important with asymmetrical lesions. It is impossible to exclude completely the action of the contralateral muscles. Fixation of the thorax is necessary particularly in patients with weak abdominal muscles and in children. The muscles are active during lateral flexion of the neck to their own side and rotation of the head to the opposite side. On flexion the position of the chin should be observed because any deviation is a sign of an asymmetrical lesion. The tip of the chin is directed towards the side of the weak flexor.

Flexion of the cervical column can take place in the following ways:

1. Maximum flexion takes place in the lower cervical and upper thoracic region. The chin moves straight forward and in the upper cervical region there is even some extension. This movement is carried out mainly by the sternocleidomastoideus.

2. Even flexion of the whole cervical region. The chin moves through an arc and moves down to the jugular notch. All the neck muscles take part in this movement although the sternocleidomastoideus only acts to a slight extent. The movement is limited by the positioning of the chin against the sternum and the length of the posterior neck muscles and the posterior ligaments.

Table 1.1

Prime mover	Origin	Insertion	Innervation
Scalenus anterior	Anterior tubercules of transverse processes C3 – C6	1st rib	Cervical plexus C5 – C7
Scalenus medius	Between anterior and posterior tubercles of transverse processes C2 – C7	1st rib, sometimes 2nd rib	Cervical plexus (C2) C3 – C8
Scalenus posterior	Posterior tubercle of transverse processes C5 – C7	2nd rib	Cervical plexus C6 – C8
Longus colli	Rectal part: bodies of vertebrae C2 – C4. Superior oblique part: anterior tubercle of atlas. Inferior oblique part: anterior tubercle of transverse processes C5 – C6	Vertebral bodies C5 – C7, T1 – T3. Anterior tubercle of transverse processes C3 – C5, T1 – T3	Cervical plexus C2 – C6 (C7)
Longus capitis	Occipital bone	Anterior tubercle of transverse processes C3 – C6	Cervical plexus C1 – C3
Sternocleidomastoideus	Sternal part: upper anterior border of manubrium sterni. Clavicular part: medial third of clavicle	Mastoid process and lateral half of superior nuchal line	Spinal accessory nerve (C1) C2, C3

Assisting muscles: Rectus capitis, muscles of the the hyoid
Neutralizers: Muscles of both sides counteract movements towards the other side
Fixators: Pectoralis major (clavicular part), subclavius rectus abdominis and lower and upper neck and back extensors

Tests for flexion

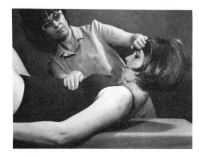

Grades 5, 4
Starting position: Supine lying.
Fixation: Light pressure from the examiner's hand on the lower part of the thorax.
Movement: Flexion of the neck with a bending forward, that is arc-like, movement. The chin points towards the jugular notch.
Resistance: With the examiner's other hand on the forehead.

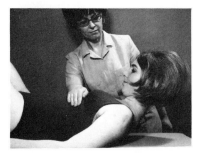

Grade 3
Starting position: Supine lying.
Fixation: The lower part of the sternum.
Movement: Complete flexion with the chin approaching the sternum.

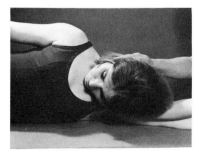

Grade 2
Starting position: Side lying with the head resting on the bottom arm and the other arm in front of the trunk.
Fixation: The head is supported on both sides in the temporal region so that the patient does not turn her head and the head and neck are in the same plane.
Movement: Forward bending of the head.

Tests for forward flexion of the head (jutting out the chin)

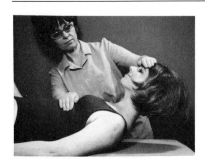

Grades 5, 4
Starting position: Supine lying.
Fixation: Slight pressure with the examiner's palm on the lower part of the thorax.
Movement: Full flexion of the neck by jutting out the chin.
Resistance: With the examiner's other palm on the forehead.

22

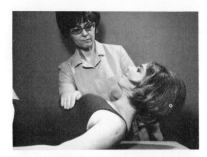

Grade 3
Starting position: Supine lying.
Fixation: The lower part of the thorax.
Movement: Jutting out the chin to the end of the range.
Resistance: Not applied.

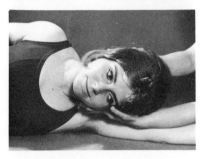

Grade 2
Starting position: Side lying with the head resting on the arm. The patient supports herself with the top arm in front of the trunk.
Fixation: The head is supported by the examiner with one hand under the cheek and the other hand on the temporal region so that the patient does not turn her head and the vertebral column is in one plane.
Movement: Jutting out the chin to the end of the range.

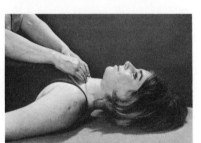

Grades 1, 0
Starting position: Supine lying.
Movement: The examiner palpates the muscle contraction at the origin of the sternocleidomastoideus and along the muscle fibres. (The other flexors are situated too deep for palpation.)

Tests for unilateral contraction

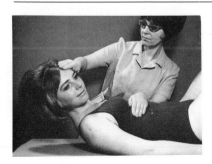

Grades 5, 4
Starting position: Supine lying.
Fixation: The palm of the examiner's hand on the lower thorax.
Movement: Flexion and rotation of the neck so that the forehead moves towards the untested side.
Resistance: With the examiner's palm on the frontal tuberosity of the frontal bone of the tested side.

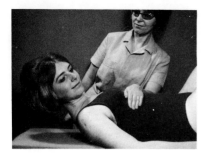

Grade 3
Starting position, fixation and movement: As for grades 5 and 4 without resistance.

Grades 2, 1 and 0 are not tested unilaterally.

Possible errors

1. On testing grade 2 the horizontal plane is not maintained.
2. In grades 1 and 0 pulsation of the carotid artery is taken to be muscle contraction.
3. Forward flexion and forward sliding are often not sufficiently differentiated.
4. Fixation of the trunk is forgotten, particularly in patients with weak abdominal muscles and in children. The necessity for fixation is clear if the patient shows a tendency to lift the lower part of the thorax from the plinth.
5. In grades 5, 4 and 3 the patient supports herself on the elbows or lifts the shoulders. The arms should be relaxed on the plinth.
6. When resistance is applied the head is pushed backwards.

Shortening

Shortening of the sternocleidomastoideus occurs fairly frequently as a congenital contracture or as an acquired torticollis after poliomyelitis or spastic paresis. Spasmodic torticollis is due to a mechanical abnormality or blockage in the vertebral column and this is not of primary muscular origin. The shortening manifests itself as rotation to the opposite side and flexion towards the same side. The deep flexors are not affected by shortening.

Note
The tests described above are not accurate enough to assess flexion in slightly weakened muscles, for example in poor posture. The muscles are considered to be of normal strength when a patient in supine lying can keep his head up (cervical spine flexed) for at least 20 seconds without effort, tremor or fatigue. This test is particularly suitable for children.

2 The neck:

Extension

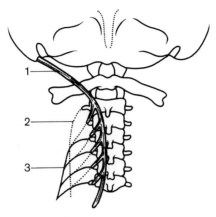

Position of the extension muscles in the neck
(1) m. longissimus capitis, (2) m. longissimus cervicis, (3) m. iliocostalis cervicis

	C1	C2	C3	C4	C5	C6	C7	C8	T1	T2	T3	T4		
		C2	C3	C4										M. trapezius
								C8	T1	T2				M. iliocostalis cervicis
	C1	C2	C3	C4										M. longissimus capitis
	C1	C2	C3	C4	C5	C6	C7	C8	T1					M. longissimus cervicis
		C2	C3	C4	C5	C6	C7	C8	T1	T2	T3	T4		M. spinalis cervicis
														M. spinalis capitis

General comments

The basic movement is extension of the neck from a position of maximal flexion with a range of movement of up to 130 degrees.

Grades 5, 4 and 3 are tested in the prone lying position with the head unsupported over the edge of the plinth. Usually both sides are tested simultaneously, although grades 5, 4 and 3 can be tested unilaterally. The movement always starts from maximal flexion of the neck. The vertebral column performs almost a continuous arc.

It is always necessary to stabilize the upper thorax, particularly in children and in patients with weak shoulder girdle or back muscles.

25

The contour of the trapezii during movement must always be observed and their symmetry assessed. Associated movements of the shoulders and extension of the thoracic region must be eliminated. It is important that the interscapular muscles especially are relaxed during the test.

The range of movement is limited by shortening or compression of the extensors of the neck and the back and by approximation of the spinous processes.

Table 2.1

Prime mover	Origin	Insertion	Innervation
Trapezius	Superior nuchal line, external occipital protuberance, ligamentum nuchae	Lateral third of clavicle, acromion tubercle on scapular spine	Spinal accessory nerve C2 – C4
Erector spinae			
iliocostalis cervicis	angles of ribs 3, 4, 5, 6	transverse processes C4 – C6	thoracic nerve C8, T1, T2
longissimus capitis	upper thoracic and lower cervical transverse processes	lateral aspect of mastoid process	C1 – C3 (C4)
longissimus cervicis	upper thoracic transverse processes	posterior tubercles of transverse processes C2 – C5	C1 – T1
spinalis cervicis	last two cervical and first two thoracic spinal processes	spinal processes C2 – C4	thoracic nerve C2 – T4
spinalis capitis	upper thoracic and lower cervical transverse processes	occipital bone	

Assisting muscles: Splenius capitis, splenius cervicis, semispinalis cervicis, semispinalis capitis, multifidus

Rotators: Rectus capitis posterior major, rectus capitis posterior minor, obliquus capitis superior, interspinales

Neutralizers: Muscles of both sides neutralize the movements at the same time

Fixators: Extensors of the thoracic and lumbar regions, rhomboidei and the inferior part of the trapezii

Tests for extension

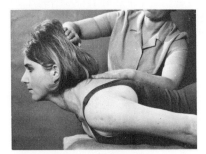

Grades, 5, 4

Starting position: The arms lie alongside the trunk and the head is unsupported over the edge of the plinth with the cervical spine in maximal flexion.

Fixation: Pressure from the examiner's palm between the scapulae and on the shoulders, and from the examiner's forearm along the thoracic spine.

Movement: Extension through the full range of movement.

Resistance: With the examiner's whole palm against the back of the head.

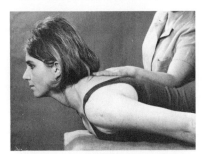

Grade 3

Starting position: Prone lying with the arms alongside the trunk, the head unsupported over the edge of the plinth and the cervical spine in maximal flexion.

Fixation: The examiner's hand and forearm between the scapulae and over the middle of the thoracic spine.

Movement: Extension through the full range of movement.

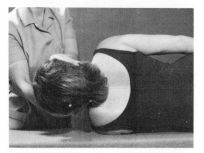

Grade 2

Starting position: Side lying with the hand of the top arm holding the edge of the plinth, the bottom arm slightly forward and the cervical spine in maximal flexion.

Fixation: The examiner supports the patient's head from below to avoid lateral deviation in the vertebral column.

Movement: Maximal extension of the neck.

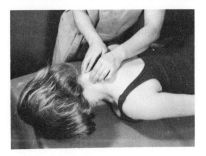

Grades 1, 0

Starting position: Prone lying. The head can be unsupported over the edge of the plinth. Otherwise it is supported on the forehead.

Movement: Both trapezii are palpated close to their origins and along the superficial muscle fibres.

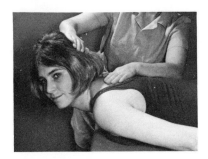

Grades 5, 4
Starting position: Prone lying with arms alongside the trunk, the head unsupported over the edge of the plinth and the neck in maximal flexion.
Fixation: The examiner's palm between and across the scapulae.
Movement: Extension of the neck with rotation towards the tested side.
Resistance: With the examiner's palm placed posterolaterally on the parietal tubercle of the rotated side.

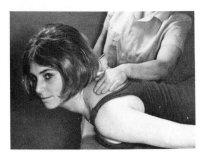

Grade 3
Starting position, fixation and movement: As above but without resistance.

Possible errors

1. When the patient contracts the muscles of the trunk, the scapulae and the shoulders, pathological associated movements are often present so that the trunk is elevated and there is an impression of motion. The arms are not relaxed and rested along the trunk and the patient supports himself on them.
2. With fixed bad movement patterns the shoulders are elevated. This always misleads to a great extent, in particular in grades 3, 2, 1 and 0. Sometimes exact assessment is impossible.

Shortening

Flexion through the full range of movement is not possible. Shortening is rarely isolated and is usually associated with shortening of the extensors of the back or with torticollis in certain conditions such as poliomyelitis, spastic paresis and various myopathies. Spasmodic shortening can exist with mechanical abnormalities of the vertebral column.

3 The trunk:

Flexion

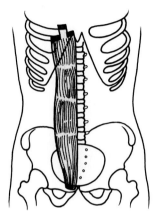

Position of the m. rectus abdominis

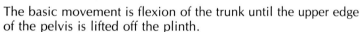

| | |T5 |T6 |T7–T10 |T11 |T12 | | | | M. rectus abdominis

General comments

The basic movement is flexion of the trunk until the upper edge of the pelvis is lifted off the plinth.

All grades are tested in supine lying. However, in grades 5, 4 and 3 the legs are bent at the hip joint at least 60 degrees, or as far as possible, to exclude the iliopsoas. If this muscle is strong then it can enable the patient to sit up by using a compensatory mechanism (*Picture* a). In such a case the patient sits up in a stiff way and lifts the trunk while maintaining or even increasing the lumbar lordosis. The abnormal movement consists mainly of flexion in the hip joint and forward and downward tilting of the pelvis. To avoid this, the trunk should be lifted slowly from the plinth so that first the cervical, then the thoracic and finally the lumbar spine is moved. The test movement is completed the instant the pelvis starts to move.

For grade 5 the position of the arms is especially important. They must be kept flexed with the elbows pointing outwards away from the head and the hands on the back of the neck during the full range of movement. The elbows must not be moved forward.

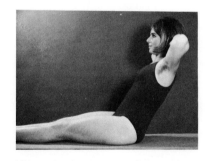

(a)

29

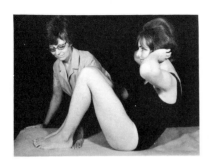

(b)

Sitting up in this way is quite hard work and so grades 5 and 4 do not need any resistance. Instead, the centre of gravity is altered through the placement of the arms. For the same reason in grades 3 and 2 the full range of movement is not expected. Grade 2 is not tested in side lying because the movement would be impossible due to friction between the trunk and the plinth. The movement of the navel must always be observed since it is drawn in the direction of movement towards the strongest quadrant. Flexion is especially great in the cervical and the lumbar spine. In the thoracic spine the degree of movement is much less and the test is concluded when the shoulder blades have been lifted from the plinth.

The fixation used in this test is not ideal, because it allows the activity of the flexors of the hip joints even if the pelvis is well fixed. If the abdominal muscles are to be differentiated more exactly then only the heels must be fixed. At the same time as flexing the trunk, the patient must increase the flexion of the already flexed knees, against resistance, without increasing the flexion in the hip joint or lifting the heels from the plinth (*Picture b*).

The range of movement is limited by the ligaments of the back, the stress on the intervertebral discs, the length of the back extensors and the movement of the thorax. A decreased range of movement from different causes is quite common and can lead to an incorrect evaluation even if abdominal muscle strength is normal.

Table 3.1

Prime mover	Origin	Insertion	Innervation
Rectus abdominis	Anterior surface of costal cartilages 5–7, xiphoid process	Pubic crest, front of pubic symphysis	Intercostal nerves 5-12

Assisting muscles: (In bilateral activity) obliquus externus abdominis, obliquus internus abdominis, psoas major, pyramidalis
Neutralizers: The muscles bilaterally counteract the tendency to rotation and side-flexion
Stabilizers: The hip flexors

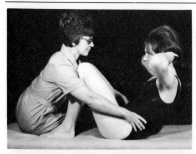

Grade 5
Starting position: Supine lying with the hands behind the neck, the hip joints bent to at least 60 degrees and the soles of the feet against the plinth.
Fixation: The pelvis is fixed by the examiner's hands. The forearms fix the legs and the feet are stabilized by the examiner sitting on them.
Movement: Sitting up with an even motion. The hands must stay behind the neck and the elbows must be kept pointing outwards. The movement is concluded when the pelvis starts to tilt forward.
Resistance: Not given.

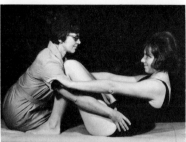

Grade 4
Starting position: Supine lying with the arms held horizontally, the hips flexed to 60 degrees and the soles of the feet against the plinth.
Fixation: The pelvis, legs and feet.
Movement: Even, slow sitting up until the pelvis starts to tilt forwards. The arms must be kept outstretched.
Resistance: Not given.

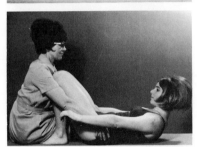

Grade 3
Starting position: Supine lying with the arms relaxed alongside the body, the legs bent and the soles of the feet against the plinth.
Fixation: The pelvis, legs and feet.
Movement: Sitting up until the lower part of the scapulae is lifted from the plinth. The arms are raised slightly.

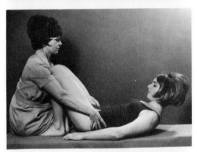

Grade 2
Starting position: Supine lying with the arms alongside the body and the legs flexed at the hip joint to 60 degrees.
Fixation: The pelvis, legs and feet.
Movement: Full flexion of the cervical spine while trying to lift the scapulae and at the same time push the lower thorax and the lumbar spine downwards against the plinth.

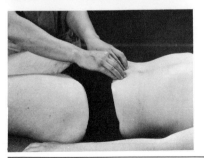

Grades 1, 0
Starting position: Supine lying with the legs in extension.
Movement: Muscle contraction is palpated in the lower part of the thorax with the flat of the hand and the fingers during coughing, maximal expiration and so on. At the same time the navel is observed. (During expiration the navel moves towards the side of the strongest muscle fibres.)

Possible errors

1. The movement is not done evenly and with the same velocity, but is jerky when the thorax is lifted.
2. At the beginning of the movement rotation of the shoulders is allowed and the exact symmetry of the movement is not retained.
3. The movement is not performed slowly and the thorax does not roll up from the plinth. A stiff action is allowed with the lumbar spine in lordosis.
4. In grade 5 a strong forward movement of the elbows occurs at the beginning of the movement. The elbows are not kept apart as far as possible.
5. The necessary flexion of the legs at the hip joints to 60 degrees is not achieved.
6. The pelvis is not fixed.
7. An excessively large movement is allowed and forward tilting of the pelvis takes place.

Shortening

Shortening does not occur.

Note

The tests described do not allow the assessment of a slight decrease in muscle strength. The abdominal muscles are considered to be full strength when the patient can sit up with 60 degree flexion in the hips while keeping the feet on the floor without any external fixation (*Picture* c). Likewise, with normal abdominal muscle strength, the patient lying supine should be able to lift the outstretched legs to about 30 degrees and circle them while keeping the lumbar spine pressed against the plinth with a slight kyphosis (*Picture* d). New electromyographic data, however, indicate that better avoidance of activity of the iliopsoas can be achieved if the curl-up is performed with extended legs and simultaneous plantar flexion of the foot against resistance.

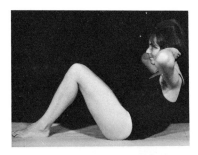

(c)

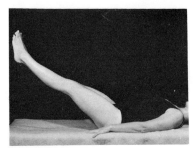

(d)

4 The trunk:

Extension (dorsal flexion)

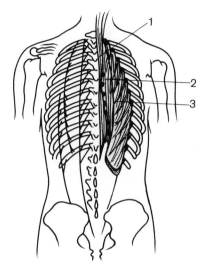

Position of the trunk muscles
(1) m. spinalis, (2) m. longissimus, (3) m. iliocostalis

			C3	C4	C5–C8	T1	T2–T10	T11	T12	L1	L2	L3	L4	M. longissimus
						T1	T2–T10	T11	T12	L1				M. iliocostalis
		C2	C3	C4	C5–C8	T1	T2–T10	T11	T12	L1	L2			M. spinalis
									T12	L1	L2	L3		M. quadratus lumborum

General comments

The basic movement is backward bending of the trunk from a slightly flexed position.

All the tests are performed in prone lying. In grades 5, 4 and 3 the thorax is kept over the edge of the plinth while in grades 2, 1 and 0 the body and the head lie on the plinth. The movement must be evaluated in two stages: during movement from flexion to the horizontal the muscles of the thoracic segment are assessed and during movement from the horizontal to maximal extension the muscles of the lumbar segment are assessed. Throughout the movement the cervical spine must be in the midposition as if it were a prolongation of the thoracic spine.

Extension of the spine is especially great in the cervical and lumbar segments and is less in the thoracic spine. In grade 2 only part of the movement is assessed. Testing in side lying is not recommended because friction of the thorax against the plinth increases the resistance and makes the movement more difficult.

Fixation must be very firm and secure.

When testing grades 1 and 0 palpation must be meticulous along the whole of the spine otherwise the muscle contraction can be missed.

The range of movement is limited by contact between the transverse processes, the facet joints and the intervertebral discs and by the length of the anterior ligaments of the spine.

Patients often complain of dizziness and so a stool on which to steady themselves should be put in front of the plinth.

Table 4.1

Prime mover	Origin	Insertion	Innervation
Erector spinae longissimus	posterior sacroiliac ligament, posterior part of iliac crest, spinal processes of the lumbar and thoracic spine, transverse processes of the thoracic and lower cervical spine	transverse processes of lumbar spine, lower ribs, posterior tubercles of transverse processes C5–C2, dorsal part of mastoid process	posterior primary rami of spinal nerves L5–C3
iliocostalis	iliac crest, upper borders of ribs 12–3	ribs 3–7, transverse processes cervical C6–C2	posterior primary rami of spinal nerves L1–T1
spinalis	spinal processes of the lumbar, thoracic and cervical spine	spinal processes (omitting an occasional segment)	posterior primary rami of spinal nerves L2–C2
Quadratus lumborum of the three or four lumbar vertebrae	Anterior part: 12th rib	Transverse processes L2–L5 of the three or four lumbar vertebrae	subcostal nerve T12, upper three lumbar nerves
	Dorsal part: transverse processes of upper four lumbar vertebrae, 12th rib	Iliac crest, iliolumbar ligament	Lumbar plexus L1 L2 (L3)

Assisting muscles: Semispinales, interspinales, rotatores, multifidus
Neutralizers: The muscles bilaterally counteract the tendency to side-flexion
Stabilizers: The hip extensors, especially in prone lying

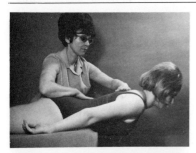

Grades 5, 4
Starting position: Prone lying with the thorax over the edge of the plinth and flexed to 30 degrees, and the arms alongside the body.
Fixation: The buttocks, the pelvis and the lumbar spine.
Movement: Extension starts in the thoracic spine towards the horizontal plane and after that maximal extension is seen in the lumbar spine.
Resistance: During the first stage with the examiner's hands between the shoulder blades. During the second stage with the examiner's hands against the lower ribs.

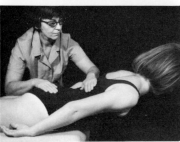

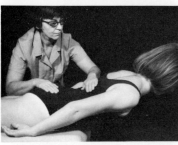

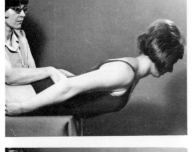

Grade 3
Starting position: Prone lying with the thorax over the edge of the plinth and flexed to 30 degrees, and the arms alongside the body.
Fixation: With both the examiner's hands on the buttocks and the pelvis.
Movement: Even back extension through the full range of movement.

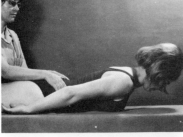

Grade 2
Starting position: Prone lying with the arms alongside the body and the thorax against the plinth.
Fixation: The buttocks and the pelvis with both the examiner's hands.
Movement: Extension of the thorax so that the head and the relaxed shoulders are moved upwards.

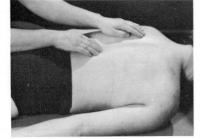

Grades 1, 0
Starting position: Prone lying with the forehead steadied on the plinth.
Movement: When the patient tries to move the thorax or at least to lift the head then the muscles are palpated carefully with the fingers along the spine.

Possible errors

1. The flexion of the thorax at the beginning of the test is not sufficient and so the range of movement is decreased and the thoracic spine is not tested properly.
2. Adduction of the shoulder blades and lifting the shoulders is allowed, and disturbs palpation of the muscle contraction in grades 1 and 0.
3. The cervical spine is not kept in the midposition in the same plane as the thoracic spine and the patient uses the trapezius.
4. Extension of both legs at the hip joint with lifting of the pelvis taking place instead of movement of the thorax.
5. Uncoordinated movements are frequent. The patient does not activate the muscles in an even manner and the contraction is not performed symmetrically and without interruption.

Shortening

This occurs frequently. It manifests itself by a change of posture. In symmetrical double-sided shortening lordosis occurs. In asymmetrical one-sided shortening scoliosis with torsion occurs and is concave towards the side of the shortening. The shortening does not always include all the muscles on one side and can be limited to one segment of the spine. This shows as stiffness of that segment and decreased movement during flexion.

5 The trunk:

Rotation

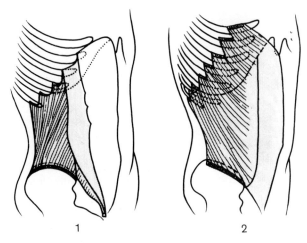

Rotational muscles of the trunk
(1) m. obliquus internus abdominis, (2) m. obliquus externus abdominis

| | | | T7 | T8 | T9 | T10 | T11 | T12 | L1 | | M. obliquus internus abdominis |
| | T5 | T6 | T7 | T8 | T9 | T10 | T11 | T12 | | | M. obliquus externus abdominis |

General comments

The basic movement in grades 5 and 4 is rotation and flexion of the trunk and in the other grades is rotation alone. The range of movement in the thoracic spine is 40 degrees and in the cervical spine is 65 degrees, of which 45 degrees is between the atlas and the axis.

All grades are tested in supine lying. Grade 2 can also be tested in sitting. Because the movement is a combined action in grades 5 and 4, the flexion and the rotation must take place at the same time and the trunk must roll up evenly without extension in the lumbar spine. The movement must take place at the same speed over the full range, without a jerk at the beginning. In grade 5 the arms must be kept apart during the full test so that they do not make the movement easier by changing the centre of gravity. In each test the arms are held in different positions: in grade 5 the hands are at the back of the neck; in grade 4 the arms

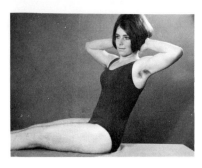

(a)

are held horizontally; in grade 3 the arms are crossed in front of the chest; and in grades 2, 1 and 0 the arms are alongside the body. For grades 5 and 4 the legs must be flexed to exclude the hip flexors as much as possible. A stiff sit-up (V-sit-up; *Picture a*) is proof of the predominance of the hip flexors.

Fixation of the pelvis is necessary even with very strong hip flexors.

During the test the position of the navel is observed. In an asymmetrical lesion the navel moves towards the strongest muscle group. In rotation towards the right all the abdominal muscles contract, but the action is relatively greater in the right obliquus internus abdominis, the left obliquus externus abdominis, the right semispinalis, the left multifidus, the left rotatores, the left latissimus dorsi and the right iliocostales. During rotation of the trunk towards the left the opposite muscles work slightly harder. Rotation mainly takes place in the cervical spine (to 70 degrees) and in the thoracic spine (to 40 degrees). In the lumbar spine rotation is almost impossible because of the position of the joint surfaces in the sagittal plane.

The range of movement is limited mainly by the location of the joint surfaces and the ligaments of the spine and perhaps a little by the obliqui abdominales of the opposite side.

Table 5.1

Prime mover	Origin	Insertion	Innervation
Obliquus internus abdominis	Deep part of lumbar fascia, anterior two thirds of iliac crest, lateral half of inguinal ligament	Anterior part of ribs 10–12, aponeurosis that splits around rectus abdominis	Intercostal nerves 7–12; iliohypogastric, ilioinguinal, genitofemoral nerves T12–L1
Obliquus externus abdominis	Eight digitations from external processes of ribs 5–12	Outer lip of iliac crest, inguinal ligament by broad aponeurosis into xiphoid process, linea alba, pubic crest, pectineal line	Intercostal nerves 5–11 (12)

Assisting muscles: In straightforward sitting rectus abdominis; in rotation iliocostales on the same side; semispinales, multifidus, rotatores, latissimus dorsi on the opposite side
Neutralizers: The ventral and dorsal muscles both counteract the tendency to flexion and extension, and the muscles on the opposite side counteract the tendency to side-flexion
Stabilizers: Obliqui abdominales, erector spinae, intercostales interni

Tests for rotation

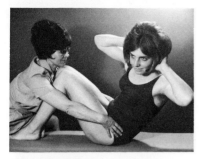

Grade 5
Starting position: Supine lying with the hands at the back of the neck, the legs next to each other and flexed as far as possible and the soles of the feet against the plinth.
Fixation: The examiner holds the patient's knees and presses them together, fixing the pelvis with the hand and sitting on the feet.
Movement: The patient performs two movements at the same time, that is trunk flexion (sitting up) and rotation mainly in the lower thoracic spine. The elbows must be kept apart as far as possible.
Resistance: Not given.

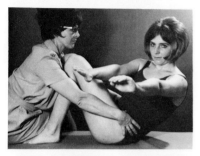

Grade 4
Starting position: Supine lying with the arms relaxed next to the body and the soles of the feet on the plinth.
Fixation: The pelvis and the feet.
Movement: Trunk flexion and rotation combined, with the arms stretched forward and moved towards the side to be rotated.
Resistance: Not given.

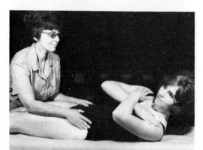

Grade 3
Starting position: Supine lying with the arms crossed in front of the chest and the legs outstretched.
Fixation: The anterior superior iliac spine of the pelvis.
Movement: Trunk rotation. While the patient turns the trunk to the side the buttocks must be kept on the plinth. First the shoulders are lifted and then the scapulae. The movement is complete when the whole of the scapula is raised from the plinth.

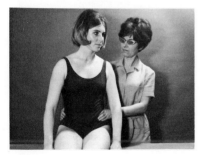

Grade 2a
Starting position: Sitting with the arms relaxed alongside the body.
Fixation: The examiner's hand on top of the anterior superior iliac spine.
Movement: Rotation of the trunk through the full range of movement.

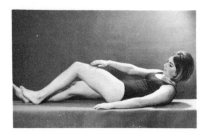

Grade 2b
Starting position: Supine lying with the arms relaxed alongside the body.
Fixation: Not necessary.
Movement: The patient lifts at the same time one shoulder and the opposite pelvis. It is permissible to stretch the arm forward and to flex the opposite leg slightly.

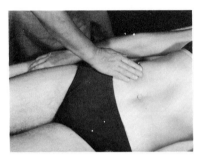

Grades 1, 0
Starting position: Supine lying with the legs outstretched. The examiner holds the patient's head slightly flexed.
Movement: As the patient attempts to rotate the trunk the muscle contraction is palpated in the obliqui abdominales.

Possible errors

1. The test is not performed with the same speed throughout. The patient tries to make a quick movement at the beginning, does not lift evenly and keeps the trunk stiff, often with increased lordosis in the lumbar spine.
2. Maximal flexion of the legs is not achieved.
3. When the obliqui abdominales are weakened, the patient tries to sit up straight and only rotates the trunk at the end of the movement by swinging the arms.
4. Simultaneous side-flexion indicates that the quadratus lumborum is taking over the movement.
5. The elbows are not kept apart as far as possible in grade 5. If they get close to each other this aids flexion or rotation.

Shortening

Slight shortening is common, but it does not limit the range of motion. It can be recognized in standing by a lateral groove along the rectus abdominis.

6 The pelvis:

Elevation (sideways lifting of the pelvis)

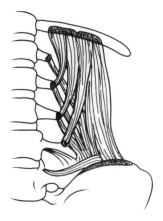

Position of m. quadratus lumborum

| | | T12 | L1 | L2 | L3 | | | | M. quadratus lumborum |

General comments

The basic movement is a raising of the pelvis. The leg on the elevated side is moved in a cranial direction so that the superior iliac spine touches the thoracic cage.

The movement takes place in the direction of the muscle fibres. Therefore the leg on the tested side must be abducted about 20–30 degrees. Tests for grades 1 and 0 are very difficult because the quadratus lumborum is situated deeply and covered by other muscles. During palpation the superficial muscles must be as relaxed as possible. Testing in standing is not recommended because standing on one leg activates a lot of muscles leading to an inaccurate result.

Fixation is not always necessary.

An informatory test of the total strength of the muscles taking part in side-flexion of the trunk is performed in side lying. The patient raises the upper half of the body sideways while the legs are fixed with a pillow between the knees to prevent pain and the pelvis is stabilized. The patient must not twist or bend the trunk forwards during the movement (*Picture a*).

The range of movement is limited because of the ribs touching the superior iliac spine and also by the spinal ligaments and the length of the quadratus lumborum on the opposite side.

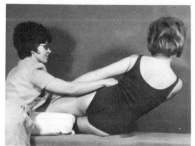

(a)

41

Table 6.1

Prime mover	Origin	Insertion	Innervation
Quadratus lumborum	Ventral part: 12th rib	Lower 3–4 transverse processes of lumbar vertebrae	12th thoracic, upper three lumbar nerves
	Dorsal part: upper 3–4 lumbar vertebrae, 12th rib	Iliac crest, iliolumbar ligament	

Assisting muscles: Latissimus dorsi, iliocostalis lumborum, obliquus externus abdominis, obliquus internus abdominis
Neutralizers: In standing: back and stomach muscles; in lying: mainly back muscles
Stabilizers: Stomach and back muscles, intercostales

Tests

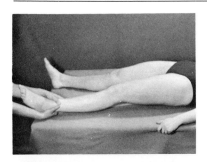

Grades 5, 4, 3
Starting position: Supine lying with the legs outstretched and slightly abducted.
Fixation: The patient holds the edge of the plinth or, if necessary, the thorax is stabilized by a second examiner.
Movement: Elevation of half the pelvis towards the thoracic cage.
Resistance: The tested leg is held above the ankle joint and drawn distally in the opposite direction to the movement. Grades 5, 4 and 3 are differentiated by the strength of the resistance.

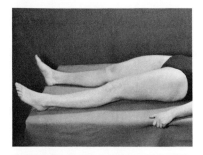

Grade 2
Starting position: Supine lying with the legs outstretched and slightly abducted (to 20–30 degrees).
Fixation: The patient holds the edge of the plinth or a second examiner fixes the thorax.
Movement: Elevation of half the pelvis in a cranial direction towards the thoracic cage through the full range of movement.

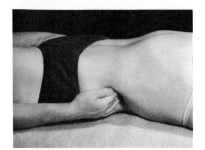

Grades 1, 0
Starting position: Supine lying with legs outstretched.
Fixation: Slight support of the tested leg below the knee.
Movement: Contraction of the quadratus lumborum is palpated next to the outer edge of the erector spinae.

Possible errors

1. Abduction of the legs is forgotten.
2. Sometimes the thoracic cage is not properly stabilized and so undesirable side-flexion of the trunk takes place.

Shortening

This causes elevation of half the pelvis and scoliosis with rotation of the spine. The scoliosis is concave on the side of the shortening. Flexion to the opposite side is decreased, especially in the lumbar region.

Part 3   The upper limb

The upper limb, and particularly the hand, is a very specialized part of the body especially so far as the unique position of the thumb and the index finger is concerned. The hand is above all an organ of grasp and as such it is capable of performing many precise and finely controlled movements. It is made up of a series of functional units which depend on each other to carry out the task of grasping. When one unit fails the whole coordination of the limb is disturbed. The vast mobility and function of the upper limb together with its great ability are only possible because of the way in which it is attached to the trunk. Mobility is facilitated by an intricate system comprising the shoulder girdle, the scapula, the clavicle and the humerus. These bones and the thorax form a complex of joints, namely the sternoclavicular, scapulothoracic, scapuloclavicular and humeroscapular junctions. In addition there is a great number of bursae, ligaments and muscle groups.

The sternoclavicular joint has features of the ball-and-socket variety, although actual rotation is of small importance. Movement of the clavicle is possible in all directions, although only to a very small degree. Isolated movement of the clavicle is of no importance but it contributes to movements of the scapula and the shoulder girdle and so increases the range of the upper limb. The main movements at the sternoclavicular joint are forward and backward motion in a horizontal plane (about 30 degrees), elevation (about 50 degrees) and depression (5 degrees).

The scapuloclavicular articulation consists of the acromio-clavicular and the coracoclavicular junctions. Anatomically the acromioclavicular joint is similar to the sternoclavicular one. Its most important movement is slight gliding rotation. The coracoclavicular connection is a syndesmosis.

The scapulothoracic connection

There are no ligaments fixing the scapula to the thorax, so that the joint is stabilized only by muscles. Scapular movements are never isolated and are associated with those clavicular movements. The scapula does not lie on the thorax in the frontal plane but forms a 30-degree angle. The scapula can rotate about a vertical axis to around 50 degrees, at which point the medial border is directed obliquely downwards and backwards and away from the thorax, during a simultaneous change of angle between the clavicle and the scapula. The position of the glenoid cavity (the socket of the shoulder joint) is dependent upon the angle of the scapula, namely the greater the angle, the more forward the movement of the socket. The scapula can carry out movements sideways (abduction) and backwards (adduction), and can be elevated or depressed. Rotation around the sagittal axis can also take place.

The scapulohumeral joint is really a double joint comprising the true shoulder joint and the humeral connection, but it always functions as a unit. The shoulder joint is a ball and socket with a small shallow socket and the small articular area of the humeral head enables a wide range of motion. Possible movements are abduction, adduction, flexion, extension, lateral rotation and medial rotation. A combination of these allows movement in many directions. Elevation of the arm takes place initially at the glenohumeral joint (up to 90 degrees) and then at the scapulothoracic articulation and the other joints of the shoulder girdle. Other factors such as posture, the bony shape of the thorax, and the suppleness of the skin and the soft cutaneous tissue are also important.

The elbow is a hinge joint between the lower end of the humerus and the upper ends of the radius and the ulna. It is divided into three parts by the joint surfaces, that is the humeroradial, humeroulnar and radioulnar articulations. The main movements are flexion and extension (0–140 degrees) and pronation and supination (0–160 degrees). A combination of these creates an increased range of motion. The ulna cannot rotate. Pronation and supination take place through the radius which only rotates around the ulna.

The structure of the hand is very intricate. It involves 29 bones: the radius, the ulna, eight carpals, five metacarpals and 14 phalanges. These permit a great variety of movements. The wrist consists of two parts, namely the proximal radiocarpal joint and the distal carpal joint. They form a functional unit and there is no independent movement. The radiocarpal, intercarpal and midcarpal joints greatly increase the mobility of the hand. The basic movements are flexion (70 degrees), extension (60–70 degrees), ulnar deviation (35 degrees) and radial deviation (30–35 degrees). Circumduction is achieved by a combination of these.

At the metacarpophalangeal joints the heads of the metacarpals articulate with the proximal phalanges. Possible movements of digits with three phalanges are flexion-extension up to 70–90 degrees, abduction, adduction and circumduction.

The interphalangeal joints are divided into proximal and distal, and are hinge joints. They can perform flexion and extension. In the proximal joints the full range of movement is up to 110–130 degrees, while in the distal joints it is somewhat less (70–100 degrees).

The thumb has only one interphalangeal joint. The carpometacarpal joint of the thumb is medially rotated and therefore the terms used to describe its movements do not have their usual interpretation. Abduction and adduction occur in the same plane as the nail, and flexion and extension take place at right angles to the thumbnail. Circumduction and rotation are also possible. A combination of flexion, medial rotation and adduction brings the thumb into contact with the fingertips, and is known as opposition. All these movements are of the utmost importance for the functional ability to grasp.

Nerve supply of the upper limb

The brachial plexus supplies the upper limb. It is usually formed from the anterior primary rami of the lower four cervical nerves and the greater part of the fourth cervical and first thoracic nerves. The anterior primary rami are the five roots of the plexus and they unite to form three trunks. Behind the middle of the clavicle each splits into anterior and posterior divisions. The three posterior divisions form the posterior cord, the anterior divisions of the upper and middle trunks form the lateral cord and the anterior division of the lower trunk continues as the medial cord.

Branches of the brachial plexus

Branches from roots:

A number of branches pass to the vertebral muscles. The C5 root contributes to the phrenic nerve.

The dorsal scapular nerve (C5) passes upwards and laterally to supply the rhomboidei and the levator scapulae. The latter is also supplied by branches of the cervical plexus. A defect of its motor function is noticeable on muscle function testing.

The long thoracic nerve (C5, C6 and C7) passes downwards behind the trunks to supply the serratus anterior. A nerve lesion is very obvious when observing the scapula because the medial border of the scapula stands away from the chest wall (this is known as a winged scapula).

Branches from trunks:

The suprascapular nerve passes through the suprascapular foramen to supply the supraspinatus and the infraspinatus. An isolated injury is very rare and a lesion causes minimal defects.

The supraspinatus abducts the humerus and it acts as a fixator when the deltoid abducts the humerus. Apart from the infraspinatus, the teres minor also acts in lateral rotation (*Picture a*).

The thoracodorsal nerve (C7, C8 and C6) supplies the latissimus dorsi and part of the teres major (*Picture b*). A slight weakening is best demonstrated by the patient extending both arms against resistance while in medial rotation.

Branches from cords:

The subscapular nerve (C5 and C6) supplies the subscapularis and the teres major. A lesion causes a weakness of medial rotation (*Picture c*).

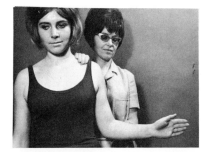

(a)

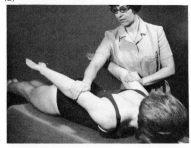

(b)

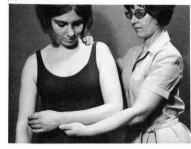

(c)

The lateral pectoral nerve supplies part of the pectoralis major.

The musculocutaneous nerve (C4–C6) supplies the coracobrachialis, the biceps brachii and the brachialis. A lesion of the nerve supplying the last two is very easy to detect. An injury of

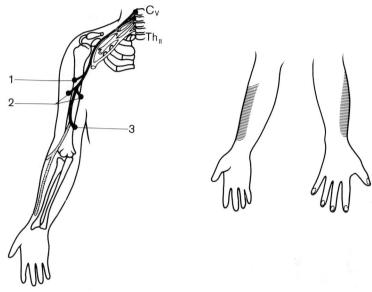

Muscle innervation sites of n. musculocutaneus
(1) m. coracobrachialis, (2) m. biceps brachii, (3) m. brachialis
The skin innervation by n. cutaneus antebrachii lateralis (= n. musculocutaneus)

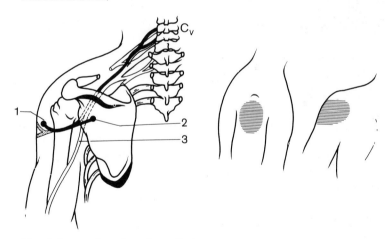

Muscle innervation sites of n. axillaris
(1) m. deltoideus, (2) m. teres minor, (3) n. radialis
The skin innervation by n. axillaris (n. cutaneus brachii lateralis)

the coracobrachialis, which in normal circumstances assists in adduction and flexion at the shoulder joint, is very difficult to detect. The musculocutaneous nerve continues as the lateral cutaneous nerve of the forearm to supply the radial side of the forearm as far as the thenar eminence.

The axillary nerve (C5–C6) supplies the deltoideus and the teres minor, and ends as the upper lateral cutaneous nerve of the arm. A lesion is mainly noticeable by the absence of deltoideus contraction. Lesions of the teres major are insignificant.

The medial pectoral nerve supplies the pectoralis minor and part of the pectoralis major.

The medial cutaneous nerves of the arm and forearm supply the skin on the medial side of the limb.

The median nerve (C6–C8, and occasionally C5) is formed by union of the terminal branches of the medial and lateral cords of the brachial plexus. It is a very long nerve and its branches supply the forearm and the hand.

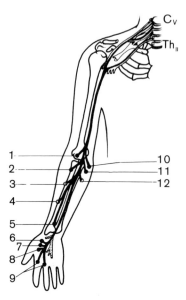

Muscle innervation sites of n. medianus
(1) m. pronator teres, (2) m. flexor digitorum superficialis, (3) m. flexor pollicis longus, (4) m. flexor digitorum profundus, (5) m. pronator quadratus, (6) m. abductor pollicis brevis, (7) m. opponens pollicis, (8) m. flexor pollicis brevis, (9) m. lumbricales manus laterales, (10) m. flexor carpi radialis, (11) m. palmaris longus, (12) m. flexor digitorum profundus

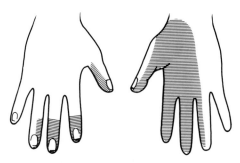

The skin innervation by n. medianus

48

The median nerve innervates all the muscles of the anterior aspect of the forearm with the exception of the flexor carpi ulnaris and the ulnar part of the flexor digitorum profundus (*Table A*). It also supplies all the muscles of the thenar eminence with the exception of the adductor pollicis and the deep head of the flexor pollicis brevis. Finally it innervates the two lateral lumbricals of the hand.

Table A
Median nerve segmental innervation C6–T1: levels of branches to particular muscles

Muscle	*Site of branch*
Pronator teres	Proximal to elbow joint
Flexor carpi radialis	Proximal to elbow joint
Palmaris longus	Distal to elbow joint
Flexor digitorum superficialis	Distal to elbow joint
Flexor pollicis longus	Proximal third of forearm
Flexor digitorum profundus (radial head)	Middle third of forearm
Pronator quadratus	Distal third of forearm
Abductor pollicis brevis	Palm
Opponens pollicis	Palm
Flexor pollicis brevis	Palm
Lumbricales manus laterales	Palm

Motor defects due to injury of the median nerve are extensive. However, many functions can be compensated by muscles innervated by the radial and ulnar nerves. Initially, the functional loss appears less than could be expected from the large area that is innervated.

A lesion of the median nerve can be detected on clinical examination by signs and symptoms and by the following tests:

1. The thumb is held alongside the index finger by the unaffected extensor pollicis longus and adductor pollicis, being unopposed by the paralysed abductor pollicis brevis and opponens pollicis. This deformity is known as monkey hand.
2. Flexion of the distal phalanx of the index finger with the middle phalanx fixed in extension is impossible due to paralysis of the flexor digitorum profundus.
3. On attempting to roll the thumbs with clasped hands there is no rolling on the paralysed side.
4. Circle test. The tip of the thumb is touched to the heads of the metacarpals. The movement is not carried out to the full range on the paralysed side, that is to the metacarpal of the little finger, but only as far as the adductor pollicis can act. The second phase, opposition, is impossible with a median nerve lesion.

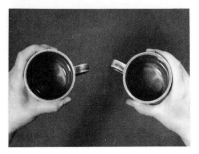

(d)

5. The 'clasped hands' symptom. The patient is asked to clasp his hands tightly. A median nerve lesion makes flexion of the thumb and the lateral two fingers impossible, and they remain extended.
6. Opposition and abduction of the thumb are impossible.
7. The mug or bottle test (*Picture d*). When a mug or bottle is gripped the pressure is less on the paralysed side and there is no contact between the mug and the web between the thumb and the index finger. This is due to weakening of abduction and opposition of the thumb.
8. Fist test. The patient cannot make a fist of the paralysed hand due to lack of flexion of the thumb and the lateral two fingers.
9. With a median nerve lesion above the branches of the nerve pronation is also affected.

Sensation is affected over most of the palm and the thenar eminence; the anterior aspect of the thumb, index finger and middle finger; part of the ring finger; and the extensor aspect and the distal half of the index and middle fingers. Due to overlap of nerves the actual sensory loss is often less. Persistent burning pain (causalgia) and trophic changes may be observed.

Table B
Ulnar nerve segmental innervation C8–T1: levels of branches to particular muscles

Muscle	Site of branch
Flexor carpi ulnaris	Proximal third of forearm
Flexor digitorum profundus (ulnar head)	Hand
Palmaris brevis	Palm
Abductor digiti minimi manus	Palm
Opponens digiti minimi	Palm
Flexor digiti minimi brevis	Palm
Lumbricales manus mediales	Palm
Interossei palmares	Palm
Interossei dorsales manus	Palm
Adductor pollicis	Palm
Flexor pollicis brevis	Palm

The ulnar nerve (*Table B*) is a long and powerful nerve which is the termination of the medial cord of the brachial plexus C8–T1. Although branches run to the forearm the main branches lie in the palm. The sensory rami of the ulnar nerve supply the dorsal and palmar side of the ulnar border, the little finger and the ulnar half of the ring finger. The motor branches innervate the small muscles of the hand, with the exception of the opponens, the flexor pollicis brevis, the abductor pollicis brevis and lumbricales manus laterales.

50

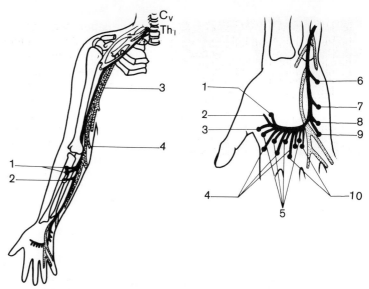

Schematic diagram of the course of n. ulnaris
(1) m. flexor carpi ulnaris, (2) m. flexor digitorum profundus, (3) n. cutaneus brachii medialis, (4) n. cutaneus antebrachii medialis

Schematic diagram of the course of n. ulnaris in the palm
(1) m. adductor pollicis, (2) connection with n. medianus, (3) m. flexor pollicis brevis, (4) mm. interossei palmares, (5) mm. interossei dorsales, (6) m. palmaris brevis, (4) mm. interossei palmares, (5) mm. interossei dorsales, (6) m. palmaris digiti minimi, (10) mm. lumbricales branch to the median nerve

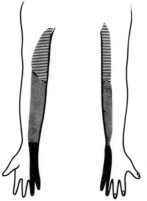

The skin innervation by n. ulnaris, n. cutaneus antebrachii medialis and n. cutaneus brachii medialis

A lesion of the ulnar nerve can be detected by clinical signs and symptoms and by the following tests:

1. The thumb is flexed at the interphalangeal joint and the ring and little fingers are hyperextended at the metacarpo-phalangeal joints, due to overaction of the extensor digitorum unopposed by the paralysed lumbricales manus mediales, and flexed at the interphalangeal joints. The index and middle fingers are less affected, due to the preserved lumbricales manus laterales. The little finger is constantly abducted to a slight extent because of the unaffected extensor digitorum. The deformity is known as claw hand.

51

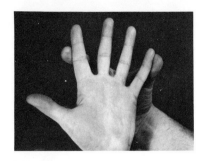

(e)

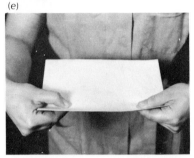

(f)

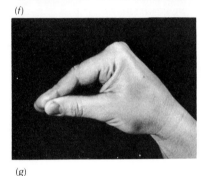

(g)

2. The patient is unable to carry out isolated adduction and abduction of the little finger with the paralysed hand (*Picture e*).

3. Test for adductor pollicis. The patient grasps a sheet of paper with both hands between straight thumbs and index fingers and tries to tear a bit off with a sudden pull. There is flexion of the distal phalanx of the thumb on the paralysed hand which is unable to grip the paper so that it is pulled towards the normal hand (*Picture f*).

4. On isolated flexion of the metacarpophalangeal joint extension is maintained in the interphalangeal joints of the index and long fingers but there is flexion of the ring and little fingers due to paralysis of the lumbricales manus mediales (*Picture g*).

5. Test of mobility of the middle finger. Ulnar deviation cannot be performed on the paralysed side because there is a sensory deficiency on the dorsal aspect of the ulnar border, the hypothenar eminence, the little finger and the ulnar half of the ring finger.

The radial nerve (*Table C*) is a terminal branch of the posterior cord of the brachial plexus (C5–C7). In the arm it has two sensory branches, namely the posterior brachial cutaneous nerve and also distally the posterior antebrachial cutaneous nerve. After the muscular rami are given off the radial nerve runs down

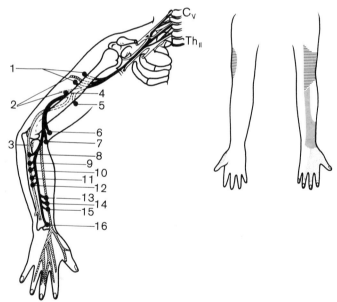

Schematic diagram of the course of n. radialis
(1) m. triceps, (2) n. cutaneus brachii posterior, (3) n. cutaneus antebrachii posterior, (4) m. anconeus, (5) m. triceps, (6) m. brachioradialis, (7) m. extensor carpi radialis longus, (8) m. extensor carpi radialis brevis, (9) m. supinator, (10) m. extensor digitorum, (11) m. extensor digiti minimi, (12) m. extensor carpi ulnaris, (13) m. abductor pollicis longus, (14) m. extensor pollicis brevis, (15) m. extensor pollicis longus, (16) m. extensor indicis proprius
The skin innervation by n. radialis and its branches

to the skin of the dorsum. This nerve contributes a large portion of the sensory supply of the arm through the posterior cutaneous nerve to the skin of the posterior and medial aspects of the upper arm, the posterior cutaneous nerve of the forearm to the skin of the posterior aspect of the forearm, and the terminal branch (the lower lateral cutaneous nerve of the arm) to the skin of the lower lateral aspect of the arm. The radial nerve supplies all the muscles of the posterior aspect of the upper arm and all the muscles of the posterior and lateral aspects of the forearm.

Table C

Muscles	Site of branch
Triceps brachii	In the proximal third of the upper arm
Anconeus	In the proximal third of the upper arm
Brachialis	In the middle of the upper arm
Brachioradialis	In the distal third of the upper arm
Extensor carpi radialis longus et brevis	In the distal third of the upper arm
Supinator	In the proximal third of the forearm
Extensor digitorum	In the proximal third of the forearm
Extensor digiti minimi	In the middle of the forearm
Extensor carpi ulnaris	In the middle of the forearm
Abductor pollicis longus	In the distal third of the forearm
Extensor pollicis longus	In the distal third of the forearm
Extensor pollicis brevis	In the distal third of the forearm
Extensor indicis proprius	In the distal third of the forearm just above the head of the radius

Symptoms of a lesion of the radial nerve are elicited as follows:

1. The forearm is pronated and there is flexion at the wrist joint and the proximal finger joints. The thumb hangs loosely. This deformity is known as wrist drop.
2. The patient is unable to clasp the hands with extended fingers due to the affected hand deviating into flexion.
3. Extension of the wrist and the metacarpophalangeal joints is impossible. Extension at the interphalangeal joints can be performed due to the unaffected lumbricales.
4. With a lesion above the middle third of the humerus the brachioradialis is also affected together with flexion at the elbow and supination of the forearm. With a lesion in the axilla, or further up, paralysis of the triceps brachii and the anconeus is added, together with elbow extension.

The sensory deficiency depends on the level of the lesion. The medial cutaneous nerve of the forearm is a long humeral nerve which supplies the anterior and ulnar aspects of the forearm. It is also a very thin nerve which serves the skin on the medial aspect of the upper arm.

The muscles of the upper limb

The most important muscles connecting the upper limb to the trunk are mainly flat muscles. They arise from the anterior and posterior chest wall and insert around the humeroscapular joint. The posterior muscles arising from the upper limb are of particular importance and are known as the spinohumeral muscles. They form the superficial layer of the muscles of the back. The muscles of the shoulder girdle run to the region of the humeroscapular joint in the following ways:

1. Inferiorly. The shoulder girdle is suspended by these muscles to a certain extent. For example, the levator scapulae, the rhomboidei and the superficial fibres of the serratus anterior and the trapezius.
2. Horizontally. For instance, the middle fibres of the trapezius and the serratus anterior.
3. Superiorly. For example, the latissimus dorsi, the pectoralis minor and the inferior fibres of the pectoralis major, the serratus anterior and the trapezius. This group has the strongest muscles.

The muscles of the shoulder girdle can also be divided into three groups by their function as follows:

1. The muscles connecting the shoulder girdle to the trunk, namely the trapezius, the rhomboidei, the levator scapulae, the serratus anterior, the pectoralis minor and the subclavius.
2. Those connecting the shoulder girdle to the upper arm, that is the supraspinatus, the infraspinatus, the teres major, the teres minor, the subscapularis, the deltoideus and the coracobrachialis. These all originate from the scapula. The clavicular head of the pectoralis major also belongs to this group, as does the latissimus dorsi, which gains a small slip of fibres from the inferior angle of the scapula.
3. The group connecting the scapula to the forearm, namely the biceps brachii and the triceps brachii.

The muscles of the forearm are mainly two-joint or three-joint muscles and the majority of them originate from the epicondyles of the humerus. Most of the flexors derive from the common flexor origin on the medial epicondyle and most of the extensors from the common extensor origin on the lateral epicondyle. They insert into the radius, the flexor retinaculum, the palmar aponeurosis and the phalanges. Their bulk generally lies close to the origin so that distally they become narrower and form tendons which run into the palm and the fingers. The thumb is unique and is dealt with separately below.

The muscles of the forearm act on the elbow, the wrist and the finger joints. When the function of the muscles is assessed the position of the elbow joint is of fundamental importance concerning both the strength and the range of movement. All the details are mentioned under each test.

The most important muscles for movement of the wrist are the extensor carpi radialis longus, the extensor carpi radialis brevis, the extensor carpi ulnaris, the flexor carpi ulnaris and the flexor carpi radialis. Although it is the only true flexor, the palmaris longus is occasionally missing and is not important. The flexor carpi ulnaris is of paramount importance and its paralysis brings about the most severe loss of flexion. The long flexors of the digits can participate in flexion at the wrist joint if the fingers are fixed. By interaction of the two extensor groups a true extension of the wrist is made possible. There is no single true extensor muscle. The long extensors of the digits can also participate in wrist extension if the fingers are fixed.

Movements of the fingers are controlled by two muscle types. The extrinsic muscles have their origins in the upper arm and the two bones of the forearm and only their tendons run into the hand. The intrinsic muscles are the inner muscles of the hand and are directly dependent on the state of the long muscles. (The thumb is again unique.) The basic movements of the fingers (with the exception of the thumb) are flexion, extension and, at the metacarpophalangeal joints, abduction and adduction.

Flexion of the fingers is ensured in many different ways because each phalanx has its own muscles. The flexor digitorum profundus acts on the distal phalanx, the digitorum flexor superficialis acts on the middle phalanx and the interossei and the lumbricales manus act mainly on the proximal phalanx. The long muscles affect all the joints they cross. However, they act only under certain circumstances. For example, the long muscles flex at the metacarpophalangeal joints with maximal power only if the fingers are extended and the wrist is held in extension. Flexion at the interphalangeal joints and the wrist almost completely eliminates the action of the long flexors.

Extension of the fingers is less well protected. It is carried out by one long muscle, namely the extensor digitorum. The index and little fingers have in addition their own extensors. The lumbricales manus also carry out extension at the interphalangeal joints, although their action is to a great extent dependent upon the position of the metacarpophalangeal joints. The function of the interossei and the lumbricales manus is not completely understood. The former are more powerful but fatigue more quickly. The lumbricales manus are weaker, but have more staying power and do not fatigue so quickly even on maximal flexion of the fingers. Their origin is displaced together with the tendons of the long flexors and so a suitable starting position is always achieved.

Adduction of the fingers is mainly performed by the interossei palmares and abduction by the interossei dorsales manus and the abductor digiti minimi manus.

The neutralizing and stabilizing functions of the muscles are to a great extent mixed in the hand and the fingers. This is shown practically in all the short muscles and the majority of the long muscles in the hand, and in the fingers with the most common movements.

The reciprocal degree of strength and the predominant activity

55

of one or the other muscle depend on the position of the arm in space and the power necessary for the particular movement. By suitable placement of the hand and careful and correct fixation it is possible to differentiate most of the muscles.

The thumb holds a unique position due to its capacity of opposition. Its range of movement is extremely wide as it has 10 muscles at its disposal. They act in the following movements:

1. Flexion at the interphalangeal joint (the flexor pollicis longus).
2. Extension at the interphalangeal joint (the extensor pollicis longus).
3. Flexion at the metacarpophalangeal joint (the abductor pollicis brevis; the adductor pollicis and the flexor pollicis longus assist after flexion at the interphalangeal joint).
4. Extension at the metacarpophalangeal joint (the extensor pollicis longus and the extensor pollicis brevis).
5. Abduction in the plane of the palm (the abductor pollicis longus and the extensor pollicis brevis).
6. Adduction in the plane of the palm (the adductor pollicis assisted by the extensor pollicis longus and the flexor pollicis longus).
7. Flexion and medial rotation at the carpometacarpal joint to 90 degrees from the palm (the abductor pollicis longus and the flexor pollicis brevis assisted by the abductor pollicis longus, and possibly the opponens pollicis).
8. External and lateral rotation to 90 degrees to the palm (the abductor pollicis longus, the extensor pollicis longus and the extensor pollicis brevis).
9. Opposition. This is a combined movement that starts with flexion and medial rotation, changes to adduction, then becomes slight flexion at the metacarpophalangeal joint followed by medial rotation of the thumb, mainly carried out by the opponens pollicis. The range of movement of the rotation is 60 degrees.

Note

Muscles that fix the scapula to the chest wall are simultaneously fixators for most movements of the arm. The number of muscles that participate and their required force is directly proportional to the position of the arm in space. To evaluate weakness in the forearm and the hand the upper limb must always be assessed. The corresponding proximal part must be fixed.

The long muscles of the hand are responsible for power and the short muscles for precision. In this respect the thumb is functionally the most important part, and paralysis of the thumb contributes to 40 per cent of the loss of function of the whole hand.

7 The scapula:

Adduction

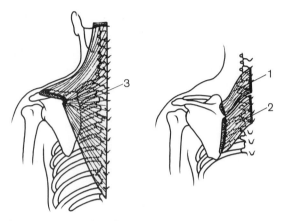

Position of the adductor muscles in the shoulder blade
(1) m. rhomboideus minor, (2) m. rhomboideus major, (3) m. trapezius

N. accessorius		**C2**	**C3**	**C4**					M. trapezius
					C4	**C5**			M. rhomboideus minor
					C4	**C5**			M. rhomboideus major

General comments

The basic movement is adduction, in which the scapula is pulled towards the vertebral column.

Grades 5, 4 and 3 are usually tested simultaneously on both sides in prone lying and with the arms alongside the trunk. Grades 2, 1 and 0 are usually tested unilaterally in sitting. The tested arm rests in forward flexion on the examination plinth. This should be high enough for the arm to be at 90 degrees to the trunk. Grades 1 and 0 can also be tested in prone lying.

Fixation of the trunk is especially important in testing grade 2. The movement is isolated to the scapula without any movement at the shoulder joint. Theoretically only the middle fibres of the trapezius carry out adduction, while the rhomboidei perform rotation as well as adduction; that is, they pull the inferior angle more powerfully towards the vertebral column. However, in practice isolation of one muscle group is not possible except with a severe isolated injury of the trapezius, when the muscle fibres of the rhomboidei can be palpated.

Resistance must be given in a correct fashion and maintained in the same direction during the complete movement. The examiner uses the whole palm because one finger can easily slip away. The index finger and then the other fingers are pressed against the scapula during the test. The range of movement is limited by the scapula touching the back muscles.

Table 7.1

Prime mover	Origin	Insertion	Innervation
Trapezius (middle fibres)	Superior nuchal line of occipital bone, ligamentum nuchae, upper thoracic spines and their supraspinous ligaments	Medial border of acromion, superior lip of scapular spine and clavicle	Spinal accessory nerve and branches C3, C4
Rhomboideus minor	Lowest part of ligamentum nuchae	Medial border of scapula	Dorsal scapular nerve C5
Rhomboideus major	Upper five thoracic spines and supraspinous ligaments	Medial border of scapula inferior to rhomboideus minor	Dorsal scapular nerve C5

Assisting muscles: Trapezius (superior and inferior fibres)
Stabilizers: The rhomboidei and the inferior fibres of the trapezius counteract each other on vertical displacement and on rotation
Fixators: Abdominal muscles and erector spinae

Tests

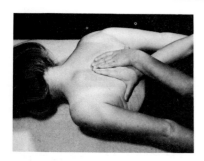

Grades 5, 4
Starting position: Prone lying with the head resting in the midposition and supported on the chin, the arms medially rotated and lying alongside the trunk and the shoulders relaxed.
Fixation: Not necessary.
Movement: The patient lifts the arms a few degrees and pulls the scapulae together with slight medial rotation of their inferior angles.
Resistance: The examiner's forearms are crossed and the index finger presses against the medial border and the thumb against the inferior angle of the scapula. The index finger reinforced by the palm gives resistance in the direction of movement.

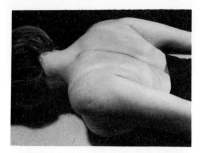

Grade 3
Starting position: Prone lying with the arms alongside the trunk and medially rotated, and the shoulders relaxed.
Fixation: It is possible to fix the lower thorax but it is not necessary.
Movement: The patient lifts the arms and pulls the scapulae together towards the vertebral column.

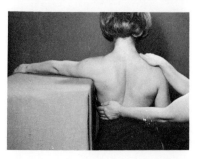

Grade 2
Starting position: Sitting on a chair beside the examination plinth. The arm rests on the plinth at 90 degrees in a position between flexion and abduction at the shoulder joint with the elbow extended and the forearm pronated.
Fixation: From behind the examiner holds the untested shoulder with one hand while the other stabilizes the thorax on the tested side.
Movement: The patient adducts the scapula by pulling the supported arm towards the body.

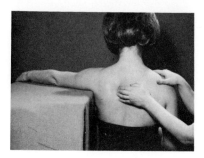

Grades 1, 0
Starting position: Sitting on a chair beside the examination plinth with the arm resting on the plinth at 90 degrees in a position between flexion and abduction. The elbow is in extension and the forearm in pronation.
Fixation: The examiner holds the untested shoulder with one hand while the other palpates the muscle contraction of the middle fibres of the trapezius between the medial border of the scapula and the vertebral column.

Possible errors

1. Frequently the patient rotates the thorax without activating the trapezius. This movement can be misjudged even as grade 2 function.
2. The resistance is neither in the correct direction nor of constant force.
3. In grades 5, 4 and 3 the patient does not use the scapular part of the deltoideus, and the scapular movement is replaced by movement of the shoulder joint.

Shortening

This is hardly ever seen.

8 The scapula:

Adduction with depression

General comments

The basic movement is adduction and inferior displacement of the scapula.

All grades are tested in prone lying. The tested arm is elevated in a sideways forwards position in order to achieve a placement corresponding to the direction of the inferior fibres of the trapezius. It is advantageous to support the arm even when the shoulder muscles are strong.

On testing grade 3, slight resistance is given in the same direction as for grades 5 and 4. Due to the position of the patient, movement against gravity cannot be tested.

The range of motion is limited by the elasticity of the superficial fibres of the trapezius, by the levator scapulae and by the interclavicular ligament. In pathological conditions it can be reduced further by contractures of the pectoral muscle.

Table 8.1

Prime mover	Origin	Insertion	Innervation
Trapezius (inferior fibres)	Spinous processes of lower thoracic vertebrae	Spine of scapula (medial border)	Spinal accessory nerve C2–C4

Assisting muscles: Trapezius (middle fibres), rhomboidei in adduction
Stabilizers: The pectoralis major counteracts adduction
Fixators: The erector spinae and the abdominal muscles fix the vertebral column, the intercostales interni and the abdominal muscles fix the ribs (particularly when the resistance is given)

Tests

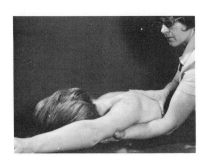

Grades 5, 4, 3
Starting position: Prone lying with the forehead resting on the plinth, the arm elevated through flexion and medially rotated, the elbow extended and the forearm pronated.
Fixation: The upper arm is supported just proximal to the elbow.
Movement: Simultaneous adduction and depression of the scapula.
Resistance: The examiner grasps the inferior angle of the scapula between the index finger and the thumb and presses it in an upward and outward direction. (The grades are distinguished by the amount of resistance given.)

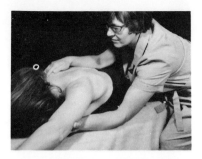

Grade 2
Starting position: Prone lying with the forehead resting on the plinth, the arm elevated through flexion and medially rotated, the elbow extended and the forearm pronated.
Fixation: The trunk. The upper arm is supported.
Movement: Simultaneous adduction and depression of the scapula.

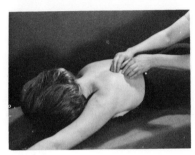

Grades 1, 0
Starting position: As above.
Movement: The muscle fibres are palpated between the scapula and the lower thoracic vertebrae.

Possible errors

1. The arm is not placed in the correct position. It is not correct to elevate the arm so that it is parallel to the head because the lower fibres of the trapezius cannot then contract in the direction of the fibres.

Shortening

This is very rare.

9 The scapula:

Elevation (shoulder elevation)

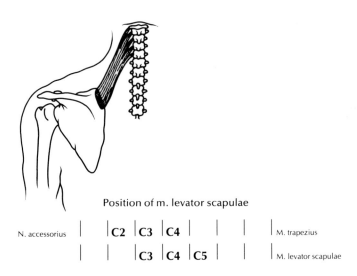

Position of m. levator scapulae

| N. accessorius | | C2 | C3 | C4 | | | | M. trapezius |
| | | | C3 | C4 | C5 | | | | M. levator scapulae |

General comments

The basic movement is elevation of the scapula.

Grades 5, 4 and 3 are tested in sitting and grades 2, 1 and 0 in prone lying. Usually both sides are tested simultaneously because a difference in strength is detected more easily this way if there is an asymmetrical lesion. The head must be observed at the same time since it remains in a neutral position with no side-flexion if the lesion is symmetrical.

The range of movement is limited by the trapezius touching the muscles of the neck.

Table 9.1

Prime mover	Origin	Insertion	Innervation
Trapezius (superior fibres)	Ligamentum nuchae (medial part), external occipital protuberance, linea nuchae	Lateral third of clavicle	Accessory nerve C2–C4
Levator scapulae	Transverse processes C1–C4	Superior angle of scapula	Dorsal scapular nerve C3–C5

Assisting muscles: The rhomboidei and sternocleidomastoideus (clavicular part) in grades 5 and 4
Stabilizers: The serratus anterior counteracts adduction, the trapezius (middle and inferior fibres) and rhomboidei counteract rotation
Fixators: On unilateral activity the lateral neck flexors fix the opposite side of the vertebral column and prevent its extension

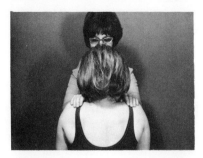

Grades 5, 4
Starting position: Sitting on a stool with the arms loosely hanging down.
Fixation: Not necessary.
Movement: The patient elevates both shoulders as much as possible.
Resistance: The examiner's palms are placed on the shoulders to press on the acromion and the clavicle.

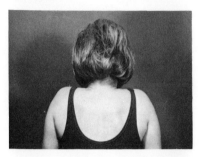

Grade 3
Starting position: Sitting with the arms hanging down.
Fixation: Not necessary.
Movement: Both shoulders are elevated as much as possible.

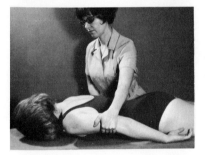

Grade 2
Starting position: Prone lying with the forehead resting on the plinth and the arms alongside the trunk.
Fixation: Slight. The examiner supports the upper arms from below.
Movement: The patient elevates the shoulders as much as possible.

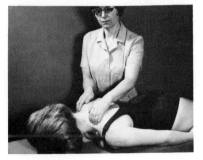

Grades 1, 0
Starting position: Prone lying with the forehead resting on the plinth and the arms alongside the body.
Movement: Contraction of the muscle fibres is palpated on the posterior aspect along the vertebral column. The clavicular part of the trapezius is palpated at its insertion on the clavicle and the levator scapulae underneath the trapezius.

63

Possible errors

1. With grade 2 occasionally it is forgotten to support the upper arms, which must not sink towards the plinth during the movement.

Shortening

This generally occurs in combination with shortening of the sternocleidomastoideus and the scaleni. Even in this context isolated shortening is very rare. It shows as elevation of the scapula and flexion of the head towards the affected side.

10 The scapula:

Abduction with rotation

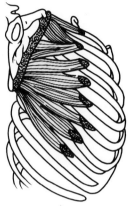

Position of m. serratus anterior

| | | | **C5** | **C6** | **C7** | **C8** | | | | M. serratus anterior

General comments

The basic movement is abduction of the scapula with slight rotation (moving the lower angle of the scapula away from the spinal column).

Grades 5 and 4 are tested in the sitting position; grade 3 supine, and grades 2, 1 and 0 sitting with upper arm supported.

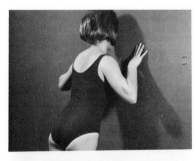

Serratus anterior (lateralis) is a key muscle in the shoulder girdle and an accurate assessment is therefore very important. A lesion of this muscle can be detected at once from the position of the scapula. On the affected side the inner edge protrudes from the thorax wall. This is scapula alata.

Serratus anterior belongs to the group of lower stabilizers of the scapula. Its examination is very important. Unfortunately the muscle function test fails in borderline cases where there is slight weakening. Here an orientation test is more suitable: the patient stands facing the wall and rests both hands against it. Then she bends the elbows and slowly brings her body towards the wall. The fixation of the scapula to the thorax wall can be observed at the same time. It is even more obvious in the press-up, particularly in the phase where the patient lowers herself to the floor.

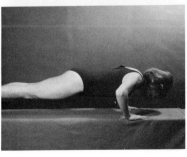

It must be emphasized that in grades 5 and 4 the thorax must be fixed.

In all grades when the arm is raised forwards it should form a right-angle or even greater angle to the trunk. The extent of the movement will be limited by the elasticity of the rhomboidei and the pars trapezoides of the ligamentum coracoclaviculare.

Table 10.1

Prime mover	Origin	Insertion	Innervation
Serratus anterior (lateralis)	With 8–9 attachments to the lateral wall of the first 8–9 ribs	Medial border of the scapula	n. thoracicus longus C5–C7 (C8)

Assisting muscles: Pectoralis major and minor
Stabilizers: Serratus anterior and pectoralis minor limit rotation on opposite sides
Fixators: Abdominal muscles, intercostales int. muscles, levator scapulae

Tests

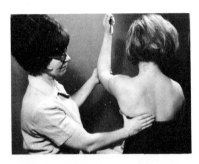

Grades 5, 4
Starting position: Seated, upper arm raised horizontally forward, elbow bent.
Fixation: With the palm of the hand the examiner holds the lateral side of the thorax under the caudal corner of the scapula.
Movement: The patient pushes the arm forward, thereby abducting and rotating the scapula simultaneously.
Resistance: The examiner's palm is placed on the elbow to counter the direction of the movement.

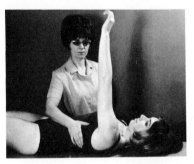

Grade 3
Starting position: The patient is supine with the arm to be tested raised vertically, and scapula supported on the plinth.
Fixation: Lateral side of the thorax, also the arm to be tested if necessary.
Movement: The patient stretches the arm forwards and upwards thereby raising the shoulder from the plinth.

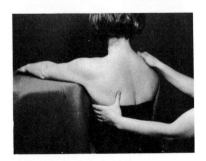

Grade 2
Starting position: Seated with the arm to be tested stretched out in front on the plinth.
Fixation: Lateral thorax wall and opposite shoulder.
Movement: The patient pushes the arm forwards and the scapula abducts and slightly rotates.

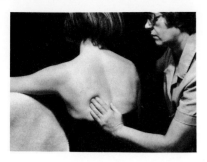

Grades 1, 0
Starting position: Seated with the arm to be tested lying stretched out on the plinth.
Fixation: Thorax if necessary.
Movement: While the patient attempts the movement a shifting of the scapula or muscle tension will be palpable on the vertebral edge of the (protruding) scapula.

Possible errors

1. Not enough importance is placed on achieving the correct scapula movement; often the examiner contents himself with a single abduction.
2. It is often forgotten that the trunk must not be rotated (this applies particularly to grades 3 and 2).
3. For grade 1, palpation must be done very carefully as part of the muscle fibre is covered by trapezius. Indications of tension can easily pass unnoticed.

Shortening

This practically never occurs.

11 The shoulder joint:

Flexion

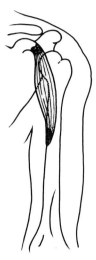

Position of m. coracobrachialis

			C4	C5	C6					M. deltoideus
					C6	C7				M. coracobrachialis

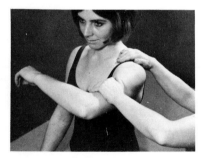

General comments

The basic movement is raising the arm forwards at the shoulder joint to 90 degrees.

Grades 5, 4 and 3 are tested in the sitting position; grade 3 lying on whichever side is not being tested; grades 1 and 0 lying supine. The movement originates from the shoulder joint. Under no circumstances should the scapula move, so it has to be fixed. The arm being tested must be rotated inwards; it is therefore best to bend it slightly at the elbow joint so the lower arm will show any rotational deviation.

Flexion of the shoulder joint is one of the movements which often produces allied movements (synkinesis): these must be carefully eliminated in the test.

The movement has no limit as it is not carried through to an extreme position.

68

Table 11.1

Prime mover	Origin	Insertion	Innervation
Deltoid (clavicular part)	Outer third of clavicle	Tuberositas deltoidea humeri	Nervus axillaris (C4), C5, (C6)
Coracobrachialis	Processus coracoideus scapulae	Mid-medial surface of shaft of humerus	Nervus musculocutaneus (C6), C7

Assisting muscles: Deltoid – middle part; pectoralis major – pars clavicularis; biceps brachii
Stabilizers: Infraspinatus; teres minor
Fixators: Trapezius, subclavius, lower scapula fixators

Tests

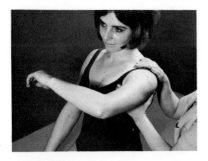

Grades, 5, 4
Starting position: Seated, arm alongside the body rotated inwards, the hollow of the hand facing backwards, elbow bent.
Fixation: Shoulder from above. The examiner stands behind the patient.
Movement: Raising the arm to 90 degrees.
Resistance: The examiner places his hand over the lower third of the upper arm above the elbow joint, the direction of the resistance changes with the arc of the movement.

Grade 3
Starting position: Seated, arm alongside the body, rotated inwards, elbow slightly bent.
Fixation: Shoulder from above.
Movement: Flexion from the shoulder joint to 90 degrees.

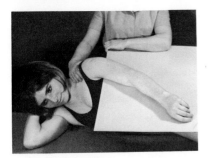

Grade 2
Starting position: Lying on the side not being tested, turned slightly backwards. The arm to be tested is rotated inwards and rests, adducted from the shoulder joint, on a smooth board which is inserted and supported horizontally between the arm and the trunk; the palm faces backwards.
Fixation: Shoulder from cranium.
Movement: Flexion from the shoulder joint to 90 degrees.

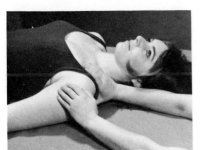

Grades 1, 0
Starting position: Supine lying, arm to be tested lying alongside the body rotated inwards. While the patient attempts movement, the examiner palpates the muscle fibres of the pars clavicularis of the deltoid on the upper surface of the shoulder joint.

Possible errors

1. If the shoulder joint is allowed to rotate outwards, the biceps brachii can substitute the movement to a certain extent.
2. The movement is not done from the shoulder joint alone — movement of the scapula and the sterno-clavicular joint is also permitted.
3. The arm deviates from the sagittal plane and combines an abduction movement. This mainly happens at the end of the movement.
4. The patient sometimes tries to substitute trunk backward bending for arm raising.
5. In the grade 2 test the board is forgotten and the arm supported by the hand only. This is not permissible as the shoulder cannot be fixed by this method and no precise evaluation can be made.
6. The board is not kept exactly horizontal.

Shortening

This rarely occurs.

12   The shoulder joint:

Extension

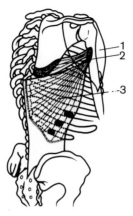

Position of the extension muscles in the shoulder joint
(1) m. deltoideus, (2) m. teres major, (3) m. latissimus dorsi

			C6	C7	C8				M. latissimus dorsi
		C5	C6	C7					M. teres major
	C4	C5	C6						M. deltoideus

General comments

The basic movement is extension at the shoulder joint in the sagittal plane 30–40 degrees backwards.

Grade 2 is tested in lying on the untested side. The other grades are tested in prone lying. The arm must be in medial rotation. Movement only takes place at the shoulder joint and the scapula remains fixed. The latissimus dorsi is a very strong muscle and therefore this test determines its function in particular. The other muscles are only of secondary importance.

The range of movement is limited partly by the flexor muscles of the shoulder and partly by contact between the greater tubercle of the humerus and the acromion process and the coracoacromial ligament of the scapula.

Table 12.1

Prime mover	Origin	Insertion	Innervation
Latissimus dorsi	Spines and supraspinous ligaments of lower six thoracic vertebrae, lumbar fascia to the lumbar and sacral spines, posterior part of the iliac crest, lower four ribs	Floor of intertubercular groove of humerus	Thoracodorsal branch of posterior cord of brachial plexus C6–C8
Teres major	Lower part of lateral border and inferior angle of scapula	Medial lip of intertubercular groove	Lower subscapular nerves (C5) C6 (C7)
Deltoideus posterior (part)	Lower lip of scapular spine	Deltoid tuberosity on lateral aspect of shaft of humerus	Axillary nerve (C4) C5 (C6)

Assisting muscles: Triceps brachii (long head), teres minor, subscapularis, pectoralis major (sternal part)

Neutralizers: Deltoideus (anterior and middle fibres), infraspinatus and teres minor all counteract primarily medial rotation

Fixators: Triceps brachii and coracobrachialis fix the shoulder, rhomboidei fix the scapula, abdominal muscles and intercostales fix the ribs, erector spinae fix the vertebral column

Tests

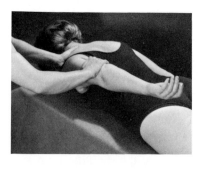

Grades 5, 4

Starting position: Prone lying with the forehead supported, the tested arm resting alongside the trunk in medial rotation and the palm facing upwards.

Fixation: Upper part of the scapula.

Movement: Extension at the shoulder joint in a sagittal plane about 30–40 degrees backwards.

Resistance: The examiner places one hand on the upper arm just above the elbow joint.

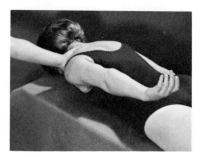

Grade 3

Starting position: Prone lying with the forehead supported and the tested arm resting alongside the trunk in medial rotation.

Fixation: Upper part of the scapula.

Movement: Extension at the shoulder joint in a sagittal plane 30–40 degrees backwards.

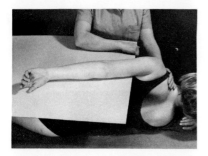

Grade 2

Starting position: Side lying on the untested side. The tested arm rests in medial rotation and some flexion on a horizontal board. The head lies on the untested arm.

Fixation: Upper part of the scapula.

Movement: The patient extends the arm to just behind the frontal plane.

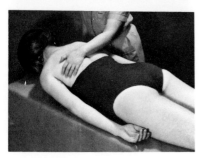

Grades 1, 0

Starting position: Prone lying with the forehead supported and the tested arm resting alongside the trunk in medial rotation.

Movement: The muscle contraction can be felt on the inferior aspect of the lateral border of the scapula. The teres major is superior to the latissimus dorsi.

Possible errors

1. The tested arm often does not remain in medial rotation during the movement.
2. In grade 2 the arm is supported not on a board but by the examiner. In this case exact assessment is impossible because the shoulders cannot be fixed and trick movements are possible.
3. Movement does not take place at the shoulder joint alone and the scapula does not remain fixed, or even moves forwards to increase the range of movement (the shoulder moves forwards and upwards).
4. When the prime movers are weak movement takes place mainly at the sternoclavicular joint. The pectoral muscles (mainly the pectoralis minor) pull the scapula into abduction.

Shortening

Flexion and lateral rotation at the shoulder joint are limited if shortening is present.

13 The shoulder joint:

Abduction

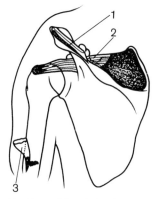

Position of the abduction muscles in the shoulder joint
(1) (origin) m. deltoideus, (2) m. supraspinatus, (3) m. deltoideus (attachment)

| | | | C4 | C5 | C6 | | | | M. deltoideus |
| | | | C4 | C5 | C6 | | | | M. supraspinatus |

General comments

The basic movement is elevation in the frontal plane to 90 degrees.

Grades 5, 4 and 3 are tested in sitting. Grades 2, 1 and 0 are tested in the supine position. The correct starting position is particularly important. It is advantageous, although not necessary, to have the elbow in flexion. The forearm then shows any deviation of rotation.

Fixation is necessary even when the muscles of the scapula are strong. The deltoideus and supraspinatus are the most important muscles of abduction at the shoulder joint. The supraspinatus fixes the head of the humerus in the glenoid cavity and enables the deltoideus to initiate movement. Thus the supraspinatus should not be ignored and even the slightest contraction should be palpated under the fibres of the trapezius.

Abduction of the shoulder joint can be performed by many substitute muscles (trick movements). The movement must therefore be carried out in a very precise manner without elevation of the scapula by the upper fibres of the trapezius. This is facilitated if the patient first depresses the scapula and flexes the head towards the tested side.

Motion is not limited in the tested range as long as there is no pathological change in the muscles or the capsule of the shoulder joint.

Table 13.1

Prime mover	Origin	Insertion	Innervation
Deltoideus (middle fibres)	Lateral border of acromion	Deltoid tuberosity of humerus	Axillary nerve (C4) C5 (C6)
Supraspinatus	Supraspinous fossa of scapula	Upper facet on greater tubercle of humerus	Suprascapular nerve (C4) C5 (C6)

Assisting muscles: Deltoideus (anterior and posterior parts), serratus anterior, infraspinatus, pectoralis major (clavicular part), biceps (long head)
Fixators: Infraspinatus, teres minor, trapezius, subclavius

Tests

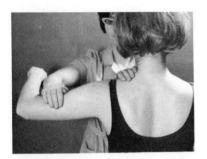

Grades 5, 4
Starting position: Sitting with the elbow flexed.
Fixation: From above on the acromion, the spine of the scapula and the clavicle. The examiner uses the whole of the hand to prevent elevation of the scapula and the shoulder. Slight rotation of the scapula is normal.
Movement: Abduction at the shoulder joint to 90 degrees.
Resistance: With the examiner's palm on the upper arm just above the elbow.

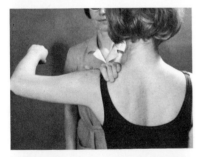

Grade 3
Starting position: Sitting with the elbow flexed.
Fixation: The scapular spine, the acromion and the clavicle.
Movement: Abduction of the shoulder joint to 90 degrees.

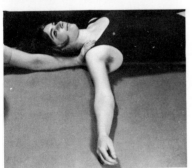

Grade 2
Starting position: Supine lying with the arms alongside the trunk.
Fixation: The clavicle, the acromion and the spine of the scapula are fixed by the examiner's palm and fingers.
Movement: Abduction to 90 degrees by sliding the arm along the support.

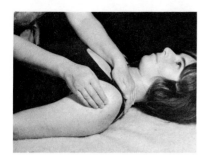

Grades 1, 0
Starting position: Supine lying with arms alongside the trunk and the palms towards the body.
Movement: Contraction of the middle fibres of the deltoideus can be palpated at their insertion on the lateral aspect of the upper arm. The supraspinatus can be palpated under the fibres of the trapezius.

Possible errors

1. The patient tries to compensate by elevating the shoulder joint (especially in grade 2).
2. The patient laterally rotates the arm during the movement in grade 2. The forearm is then supinated and the long head of the biceps brachii and the anterior fibres of the deltoideus act as substitutes.
3. The trunk is bent to the opposite side.

Shortening

This is very rare except after a long fixation of the arm in abduction.

14 The shoulder joint:

Extension from abduction

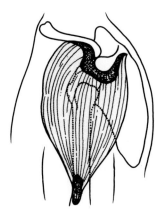

Position of m. deltoideus

| | | C_4 | C_5 | C_6 | | | | M. deltoideus

General comments

In the basic movement, from a starting position of 90 degrees flexion, the upper arm is moved sideways and backwards in a horizontal plane. The whole range of motion is 120 degrees, but in grades 5, 4 and 3 only the last 20–30 degrees are included.

The range of movement is mainly limited by the anterior structures of the capsule of the shoulder joint.

Table 14.1

Prime mover	Origin	Insertion	Innervation
Deltoideus (posterior fibres)	Scapular spine	Deltoid tuberosity of humerus	Axillary nerve (C4) C5 (C6)

Assisting muscles: Infraspinatus, teres minor, latissimus dorsi
Stabilizers: Deltoideus (middle part) and supraspinatus counteract latissimus dorsi and teres minor. The adduction component of infraspinatus and teres minor counteracts rotation
Fixators: Trapezius and rhomboidei fix the scapula

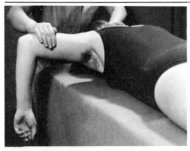

Grades 5, 4
Starting position: Prone lying with the forehead supported. The tested arm is in 90-degree abduction at the shoulder joint and 90-degree flexion at the elbow joint.
Fixation: The scapula is fixed on the spine.
Movement: Extension.
Resistance: On the upper arm just above the elbow.

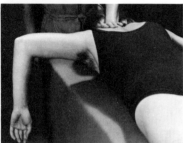

Grade 3
Starting position: Prone lying with the forehead supported. The test arm is abducted at the shoulder joint and flexed at the elbow joint.
Fixation: The scapula and the lateral thorax.
Movement: Extension of the upper arm.

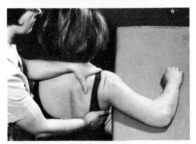

Grade 2
Starting position: Sitting on a stool with the test arm resting on a plinth in 90-degree flexion and slight abduction at the shoulder joint and flexed to 90 degrees at the elbow joint.
Fixation: The scapula and the lateral aspect of the thorax.
Movement: The full range of movement from the starting position.

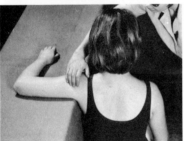

Grades 1, 0
Starting position: Sitting with the test arm resting on a plinth in a position between flexion and abduction. The elbow is flexed.
Movement: The fibres of the posterior part of the deltoideus can be palpated on the posterior part of the shoulder.

Possible errors

1. The movement is not performed at the shoulder joint.
2. The patient replaces or assists the movement by adduction of the shoulder or rotation of the trunk.
3. When the movement is attempted with the triceps brachii, the elbow extends.

Shortening

This is very rare.

15 The shoulder joint:

Flexion from abduction

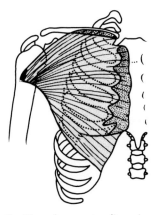

Position of m. pectoralis major

		C5	C6								M. pectoralis major - pars clavicularis
			C6	C7							M. pectoralis major – pars sternocostalis
					C8	T1					M. pectoralis major – pars abdominalis

General comments

In the basic movement, from a position of abduction the upper arm is moved forwards in a horizontal plane to a position of pure flexion. The range of movement is 120–130 degrees.

Grades 5, 4 and 3 are tested in supine lying. Grades 2, 1 and 0 are tested in sitting with the test arm supported. The plinth must be high enough for the arm to be at 90 degrees to the trunk. By activating the whole of the pectoralis major the resulting movement is pure adduction. When testing grades 5, 4 and 3 it is possible to some extent to distinguish between the clavicular and sternocostal parts of the muscle by changing the starting position and the direction of resistance. These should encourage the maximal response from the tested muscles. The fibres of the clavicular head run downwards and so to test them the arm must be at an acute angle to the trunk, preferably about 70 degrees. The fibres of the sternocostal head run horizontally and upwards, and to test them, the arm must be at an obtuse angle to the trunk and preferably at about 110 degrees.

The range of movement is limited by the thorax.

Table 15.1

Prime mover	Origin	Insertion	Innervation
Pectoralis major	Clavicular part: medial half of anterior surface of clavicle	Lateral lip of intertubercular groove of humerus	Lateral and medial thoracic nerves C5, C6, C7
	Sternocostal part: anterior surface of sternum, upper six costal cartilages Abdominal part: upper part of external oblique aponeurosis		Abdominal part C8, T1

Assisting muscles: Deltoideus (anterior part), coracobrachialis
Stabilizers: None
Fixators: The upper fibres of the trapezius and perhaps also the subclavius help to fix the clavicle; the serratus anterior and the middle fibres of the trapezius fix the scapula

Tests

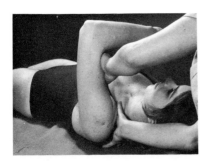

Grades 5, 4
Starting position: Supine lying with the arm in abduction at the shoulder joint, flexion at the elbow and with the forearm and fingers directed upwards toward the ceiling.
Fixation: The shoulder.
Movement: The patient moves the arm forwards 90 degrees.
Resistance: On the upper arm just above the elbow.
N.B. The picture illustrates the end of the range.

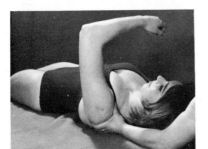

Grade 3
Starting position: Supine lying with the arm in abduction at the shoulder joint and with flexion at the elbow.
Fixation: The shoulder.
Movement: To flexion of the shoulder joint.

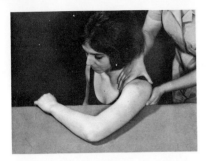

Grade 2
Starting position: Sitting with the arm resting in abduction to 90 degrees on the plinth and the palm facing downward.
Fixation: The scapula and the lateral aspect of the thorax.
Movement: The arm slides forward on the support through the full range of movement to a position of flexion.

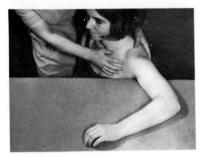

Grades 1, 0
Starting position: Sitting with the arm resting in abduction to 90 degrees at the shoulder joint, with flexion at the elbow, and with the palm facing downwards.
Movement: The muscle fibres can be palpated close to their insertion on the intertubercular groove, along their course on the anterior aspect of the thorax, and on the anterior fold of the axilla.

Possible errors

1. The patient often tries to carry out the movement with the assistance of the upper part of the trapezius or by contraction of all the muscles of the shoulder girdle.
2. In grades 5 and 4 the patient often tries to overcome the resistance by stronger flexion of the elbow joint (biceps brachii). It is necessary to maintain the same position at the elbow joint, that is, flexion.

Shortening

With shortening the range of movement of extension from abduction at the shoulder joint is reduced. The shoulder is protracted and the scapula is abducted.

81

16 The shoulder joint:

Lateral rotation

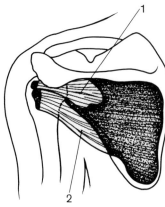

Muscles of lateral rotation
(1) m. infraspinatus, (2) m. teres minor

		C4	C5	C6						M. infraspinatus
		C4	C5	C6						M. teres minor

General comments

The basic movement is lateral rotation at the shoulder joint. The test is carried through a range of movement of 90 degrees.

All grades are examined in prone lying. With grades 5, 4 and 3 the arm is abducted to 90 degrees at the shoulder joint, the upper arm rests on the plinth and the forearm hangs down over the edge of the plinth. In grades 2, 1 and 0 the whole arm hangs down and is flexed at the shoulder joint to 90 degrees. The middle fibres of the deltoideus often assist movement. In grades 5, 4 and 3 the trapezius is activated as a fixator. When the patient finds difficulty in relaxing the deltoideus and is unable to relax the trapezius despite correct positioning of the head and neck, it is better to perform the test in supine lying. In this position the arm is slightly abducted at the shoulder joint and flexed at the elbow. If the test is carried out in this manner, the fact must be recorded on the assessment card.

It is recommended to put either the examiner's hand with the palm facing upwards or a small cushion between the arm and the edge of the plinth since occasionally patients complain of pain from the pressure of the edge.

Fixation of the scapula is necessary with children and patients with weak deltoidei.

The range of movement is limited by the muscles of medial rotation, the coracohumeral ligament and the joint capsule.

Table 16.1

Prime mover	Origin	Insertion	Innervation
Infraspinatus	Medial two thirds of infraspinous fossa of scapula	Middle facet of greater tubercle of humerus	Suprascapular nerve (C4) C5 (C6)
Teres minor	Upper two thirds of lateral border of scapula	Lower facet of greater tubercle of humerus	Axillary nerve, often branches of suprascapular nerve (C4) C5 (C6)

Assisting muscles: Deltoideus (posterior part)
Stabilizers: None
Fixators: Trapezius (middle part) and rhomboidei fix the scapula

Tests

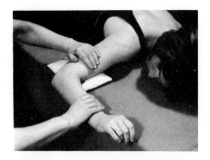

Grades 5, 4
Starting position: Prone lying with the head rotated towards the tested side. The arm is supported and abducted to 90 degrees at the shoulder joint and flexed to 90 degrees at the elbow. The forearm hangs over the edge of the plinth and the elbow rests on a small pillow.
Fixation: Slight pressure on the upper arm just above the elbow so as not to interfere with the movement. If necessary the scapula may be fixed with pressure over its spine.
Movement: The shoulder is rotated laterally through the full range of movement. The forearm moves forward and upward. At the end of the range the palm should be facing the floor and the forearm should be horizontal.
Resistance: With the palm on the forearm just above the wrist joint.

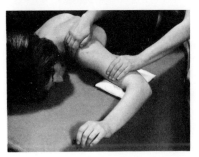

Grade 3
Starting position: Prone lying with the head rotated towards the tested side. The upper arm is supported and abducted to 90 degrees at the shoulder joint. The forearm hangs over the edge of the plinth and the elbow rests on a small pillow.
Fixation: The scapula and the upper arm just above the elbow joint.
Movement: The shoulder is rotated laterally through the full range of movement. The forearm moves from a vertical to a horizontal position and at the end of the range the palm should face the floor.

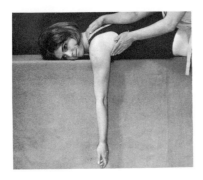

Grade 2
Starting position: Prone lying close to the edge of the plinth with the head rotated toward the tested side. The arm hangs over the edge of the plinth and is medially rotated at the shoulder joint.
Fixation: The scapula is fixed by the examiner with one hand on its spine and the other on the lateral border of the scapula.
Movement: The shoulder is rotated laterally through the full range of movement.

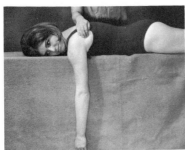

Grades 1, 0
Starting position: Prone lying with the head rotated toward the tested side. The arm is medially rotated and hangs over the edge of the plinth.
Movement: The teres minor is carefully palpated on the superior aspect of the lateral border of the scapula. The infraspinatus is palpated just above.

Possible errors

1. With grades 5, 4 and 3 the muscles of the forearm, wrist and hand do not remain relaxed.
2. In grades 5, 4 and 3 if the resistance is too great, the patient may try to extend the elbow and the wrist.
3. In grade 2 the movement does not take place at the shoulder joint.

Shortening

This is very rare and causes the upper arm to be laterally rotated.

17 The shoulder joint:

Medial rotation

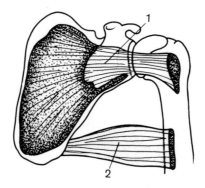

Muscles of medial rotation
(1) m. subscapularis, (2) m. teres major

		C5	C6	C7	C8				M. subscapularis
		C5	C6						M. pectoralis major – pars clavicularis
			C6	C7					M. pectoralis major – pars sternocostalis
					C8	T1			M. pectoralis major – pars abdominalis
			C6	C7	C8				M. latissimus dorsi
		C5	C6	C7					M. teres major

General comments

The basic movement is medial rotation at the shoulder joint with a range of 90 degrees.

All grades are tested in prone lying. With grades 5, 4 and 3 the arm is abducted to 90 degrees at the shoulder joint and the forearm hangs down over the edge of the plinth. In grades 2, 1 and 0 the whole arm hangs over the edge of the plinth in lateral rotation.

The necessity for fixation depends on the strength of the muscles of the shoulder girdle and their own capacity for fixation. As in lateral rotation it is advantageous to support the elbow on the edge of the plinth with a small pillow or with the hand.

The range of movement is limited by the joint capsule and by the muscles of lateral rotation.

Table 17.1

Prime mover	Origin	Insertion	Innervation
Subscapularis	Medial three quarters of costal surface of scapula	Lesser tubercle of humerus	Upper and lower subscapular nerve C5, C6, (C7) (C8)
Pectoralis major	Clavicular part: medial half of anterior surface of clavicle Sternocostal part: anterior surface of sternum, upper six costal cartilages Abdominal part: upper part of external oblique aponeurosis	Lateral lip of intertubercular groove	Lateral and medial thoracic nerves C5, C6 C6, C7 C8, T1
Latissimus dorsi	Spinal part: spines and supraspinatous ligaments of lower six thoracic vertebrae Costal part: by the lumbar fascia to the lumbar and sacral vertebral spines Pelvic part: posterior part of iliac crest, lower four ribs	Floor of intertubercular groove	Thoracodorsal nerve C6–C8
Teres major	Inferior angle and lower part of lateral border of scapula	Medial lip of intertubercular groove	Lower subscapular nerve (C5) C6 (C7)

Assisting muscles: Deltoideus (anterior part), biceps brachii, coracobrachialis
Stabilizers: Deltoideus (anterior part), coracobrachialis and pectoralis (clavicular head) counteract the extension of latissimus dorsi and teres major
Fixators: Pectoralis major and serratus anterior fix the scapula

Tests

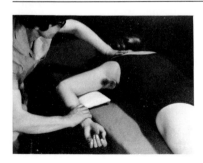

Grades 5, 4
Starting position: The arm is abducted to 90 degrees at the shoulder joint and flexed to 90 degrees at the elbow. The forearm hangs over the edge of the plinth and the elbow rests on a small pillow.
Fixation: Slight pressure with the examiner's hand just above the elbow. If necessary, the spine of the scapula can also be fixed.
Movement: The shoulder is rotated medially through the full range of movement. The forearm moves backward and upward through 90 degrees (so that at the end of the range the palm faces the ceiling).
Resistance: With the examiner's palm against the forearm just above the wrist joint.

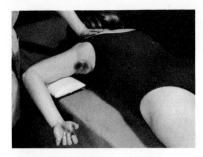

Grade 3

Starting position: Prone lying with the arm abducted to 90 degrees at the shoulder joint. The forearm hangs over the edge of the plinth and the elbow rests on a small pillow.

Fixation: Either the upper arm alone, just above the elbow, or the scapula as well. The latter is necessary when the muscles of the shoulder girdle are weak.

Movement: Medial rotation at the shoulder joint through the full range of movement.

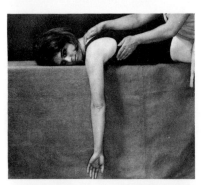

Grade 2

Starting position: Prone lying close to the edge of the plinth with the arm hanging over the edge and laterally rotated at the shoulder joint and extended at the elbow.

Fixation: The scapula and the clavicle.

Movement: Medial rotation at the shoulder joint through the full range of movement.

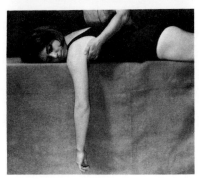

Grades 1, 0

Starting position: Prone lying close to the edge of the plinth. The arm is hanging in lateral rotation.

Movement: The subscapularis muscle can be palpated deep in the axilla close to its insertion. However, it is very difficult to establish a contraction because of the localization. The latissimus dorsi and the teres major can be palpated on the posterior fold of the axilla, and the pectoralis major on the anterior fold.

Possible errors

1. The muscles of the hand and the wrist are not relaxed in grades 5, 4 and 3.
2. Flexion of the elbow is not 90 degrees.
3. If the pectoralis major predominates, there is a tendency for adduction to occur.

Shortening

The arm is medially rotated if shortening is present. In supine lying the patient is unable to elevate the arm fully to rest it on the plinth alongside the head.

18 The elbow joint:

Flexion

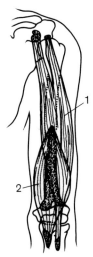

Flexion muscles in the elbow
(1) m. biceps brachii, (2) m. brachialis

			C5	C6						M. biceps brachii
			C5	C6						M. brachialis
			C5	C6						M. brachioradialis

General comments

The basic movement is flexion at the elbow joint with a range of movement of 150 degrees.

Grades 5, 4 and 3 are tested in sitting, grade 2 is tested in lying and sitting and grades 1 and 0 are tested in supine lying.

The position of the forearm and the hand is particularly important during this test. Flexion of the elbow is a movement of the greatest importance to the human being, and so this function is guaranteed by a large number of muscles each of which is activated to a different degree depending upon the placement of the forearm. Supination of the forearm is most favourable for the biceps brachii and is used as a basic position. Examination of flexion at the elbow joint starts from this point. The brachioradialis works most effectively when the forearm is midway between pronation and supination. The brachialis participates to the greatest degree when the forearm is pronated, as does the pronator teres. The brachialis is activated during flexion with all positions of rotation of the forearm. The brachioradialis constitutes a reserve of strength mainly utilized in movements against resistance.

Other muscles that participate in flexion of the elbow are the long flexors of the hand and the fingers, which originate from the epicondyles of the humerus. The most important are the flexor carpi radialis, the flexor carpi ulnaris, the extensor carpi radialis longus, the extensor carpi radialis brevis, the palmaris longus and the flexor digitorum superficialis. If these muscles are activated too strongly during an attempt to carry out elbow flexion, the position of the fingers and the wrist is altered.

During flexion, in particular against resistance, there is a tendency for hyperextension at the shoulder joint to occur. To prevent this, the elbow must be fixed slightly without limiting the movement.

On testing it must be remembered that the biceps brachii is the most important flexor. Differentiation of the muscles is a well-established means of deciding on future treatment and the arm should be positioned so that the biceps brachii can act as the principal flexor. If this fails then the brachioradialis should be strengthened to become the main flexor. A slight weakness of the biceps brachii only shows on testing if the movement starts from maximal extension.

Slight weakening is best shown when the movement (especially against resistance) is performed from hyperextension (*Picture a*) to 4 degrees of flexion (*Picture b*). This starting position is very unsuitable for the muscle because it demands immediate activity at full strength.

The range of movement is limited by the coronoid process of the ulna articulating with the coronoid fossa of the humerus, and by compression of the muscles of the upper arm and the forearm.

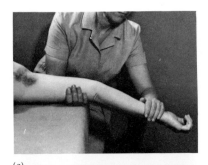

(a)

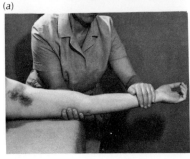

(b)

Table 18.1

Prime mover	Origin	Insertion	Innervation
Biceps brachii	Long head: supraglenoid tubercle of scapula Short head: tip of coracoid process	Radial tuberosity of radius Bicipital aponeurosis into deep fascia over medial aspect of forearm and posterior border of ulna	Musculocutaneous nerve C5 C6
Brachialis	Distal half of anterior surface of humerus, medial intermuscular septum	Anterior surface of coronoid process of ulna	Musculocutaneous nerve C5 C6 A few fibres from radial nerve
Brachioradialis	Upper two thirds of lateral supracondylar ridge of humerus	Lateral aspect of lower end of radius	Radial nerve C5 C6

Assisting muscles: Flexor carpi radialis, flexor carpi ulnaris, extensor carpi ulnaris, extensor carpi radialis longus, palmaris longus, pronator teres
Stabilizers: Pronator teres and biceps brachii counteract each other's rotation
Fixators: Pectoralis major, deltoideus (anterior part) and coracobrachialis fix the humerus in a vertical position

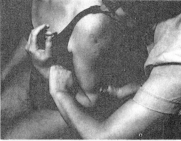

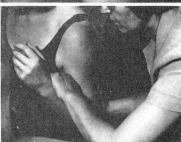

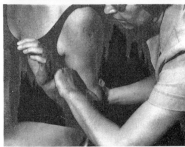

Grades 5, 4

Starting position: Sitting with the tested arm alongside the trunk. The forearm is in supination for the biceps brachii, midposition for the brachioradialis and pronation for the brachialis.

Fixation: Posterior aspect of the upper arm just above the elbow, leaving the joint free to move.

Movement: Flexion of the elbow with the full range of movement.

Resistance: On the forearm just above the wrist. The forearm remains in the same position throughout the movement.

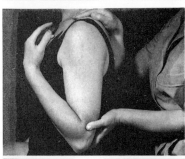

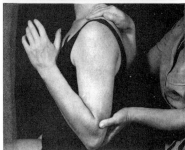

Grade 3

Starting position: Sitting with the arm alongside the trunk. The forearm is in supination for the biceps brachii, in the midposition for the brachioradialis and in pronation for the brachialis.

Fixation: The examiner grasps the posterior aspect of the elbow with one hand while the other fixes the shoulder and the scapula as necessary.

Movement: Flexion of the elbow through the full range of movement. The forearm remains in the same position throughout.

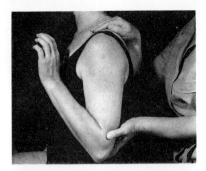

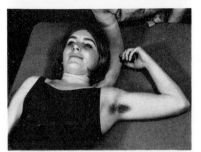

Grade 2a
Starting position: Supine lying with the upper arm abducted to 90 degrees, with lateral rotation at the shoulder joint and with extension at the elbow. The forearm rests on the plinth on the radial border for the biceps brachii, on the posterior aspect for the brachioradialis and on the ulnar border for the brachialis.
Fixation: The shoulder and the epicondyles of the elbow if necessary.
Movement: Flexion of the elbow through the full range of movement by sliding the forearm on the support.

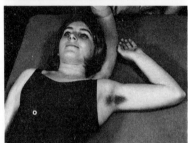

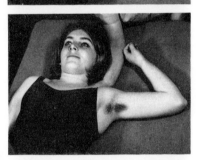

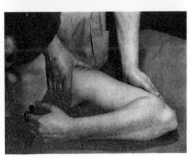

Grade 2b
Starting position: Sitting with the tested side towards the plinth. The arm is abducted to 90 degrees at the shoulder and extended at the elbow. The forearm rests on the plinth on the ulnar border for the biceps brachii, on the anterior aspect for the brachioradialis and on the radial border for the brachialis.
Fixation: The middle third of the upper arm and the shoulder.
Movement: Flexion of the elbow through the full range of movement by sliding the forearm on the support.

91

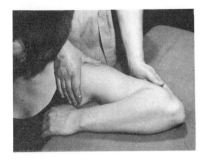

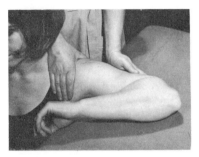

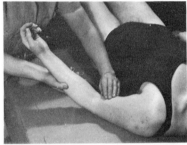

Grades 1, 0

Starting position: Supine with the arm slightly abducted and laterally rotated at the shoulder joint and the elbow slightly flexed. The forearm is in supination for the biceps brachii, in midposition for the brachioradialis and in pronation for the brachialis.

Movement: The tendon of the biceps brachii can be palpated in the fold of the elbow close to its insertion and the muscle fibres can be palpated along their course on the anterior aspect of the upper arm. The brachioradialis can be palpated close to its origin along the muscle fibres. The brachialis can be palpated over the coronoid process of the ulna and along the course of the muscle fibres on the lateral aspect of the lower third of the humerus.

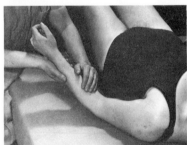

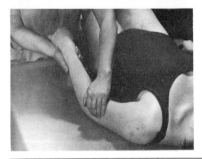

Possible errors

Mistakes are often made.
1. The starting positions are not observed exactly and the movements are assessed as a whole.
2. The activity of the flexors of the wrist is ignored. When these muscles assist the movement in supination, wrist flexion takes place simultaneously with elbow flexion.
3. In the same fashion the activity of the wrist extensors is not observed. If they assist during flexion of the elbow in pronation, there is extension of the wrist.
4. Correct fixation of the elbow is not observed. The joint must remain free.
5. The test does not start from full extension of the elbow.

Shortening

This shows as a position of flexion to a varying degree, depending on its extent.

19   The elbow joint:

Extension

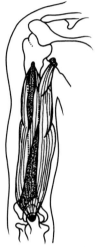

Position of m. triceps brachii

|	|	C6	C7	C8	|	|	|	|		M. triceps brachii – caput longum
|	|	C6	C7		|	|	|	|		M. triceps brachii – caput laterale
|	|	|	C7	C8	|	|	|	|		M. triceps brachii – caput mediale
|	|	|	C7	C8	|	|	|	|		M. anconeus

General comments

The basic movement is extension at the elbow joint with a range of 90 degrees.

Grades 5, 4 and 3 are tested in prone lying. The arm is abducted at the shoulder joint and the forearm hangs over the edge of the plinth. For grade 2 the starting position is supine lying or sitting. In grades 1 and 0 the starting position is supine lying. Where the arm rests over the edge of the plinth, the elbow is supported by the hand of the examiner or by a small pillow. The examiner's hand may gently fix the arm.

The main extensor of the elbow is the triceps brachii. The action of the anconeus is often disregarded although the strength of extension may be reduced by about 20 per cent in an isolated injury of this muscle. In doubtful cases it is therefore valuable to palpate contraction of the anconeus (test grade 1) behind the lateral epicondyle of the humerus.

The range of movement is limited by the articulation of the olecranon of the ulna in the olecranon fossa of the humerus.

Table 19.1

Prime mover	Origin	Insertion	Innervation
Triceps brachii	Long head: infraglenoid tubercle of scapula	Olecranon of ulna	Radial nerve C6 C7 C8
	Lateral head: a linear attachment from upper border of radial groove of humerus		C6 C7
	Medial head: whole posterior surface of humerus below radial groove, adjacent medial and lateral intermuscular septa		C7 C8
Anconeus	Lateral epicondyle of humerus, radial collateral ligament	Lateral surface of olecranon of ulna, posterior surface of ulna	Radial nerve C7 C8

Assisting muscles: Extensors of the forearm
Stabilizers: None
Fixators: Pectoralis major (sternal part), latissimus dorsi, teres major

Tests

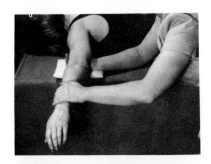

Grades 5, 4
Starting position: Prone lying with the arm abducted to 90 degrees at the shoulder joint. The forearm hangs over the edge of the plinth. The elbow is at 90 degrees.
Fixation: The examiner's palm fixes the anterior aspect of the upper arm just above the elbow.
Movement: Extension of the elbow to the end of the range.
Resistance: With the examiner's hand on the posterior aspect of the forearm just above the wrist.

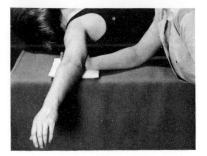

Grade 3
Starting position: Prone lying with the arm abducted to 90 degrees at the shoulder joint. The forearm hangs over the edge of the plinth and the elbow is at 90 degrees.
Fixation: The examiner's palm on the anterior aspect of the upper arm just above the elbow.
Movement: Extension of the elbow.

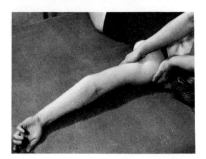

Grade 2a
Starting position: Supine lying. The arm rests on the plinth and is abducted to 90 degrees and laterally rotated at the shoulder joint. The forearm is in supination and flexed to 90 degrees at the elbow.
Fixation: The upper arm and shoulder girdle.
Movement: Extension of the elbow so that the forearm moves over the support.

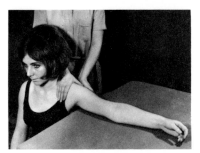

Grade 2b
Starting position: Sitting with the tested side next to the plinth. The arm rests on the plinth abducted to 90 degrees at the shoulder joint, the forearm is in the midposition (the hand rests on the ulnar border and the elbow is flexed to 90 degrees).
Fixation: The upper arm and the shoulder girdle.
Movement: The forearm slides over the plinth and the elbow extends.

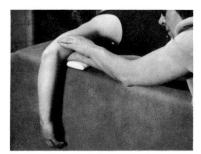

Grades 1, 0
Starting position: Prone lying with the arm abducted at the shoulder joint. The forearm hangs over the edge of the plinth.
Movement: The tendon of the triceps brachii can be palpated at its insertion on the posterior aspect of the elbow. The muscle fibres can be palpated along their course on the upper arm. The anconeus can be palpated behind the lateral epicondyle of the humerus.

Possible errors

These are rare.

Shortening
If there is shortening then flexion is difficult at the elbow joint and there is a reduced range of movement.

20 The forearm:

Supination

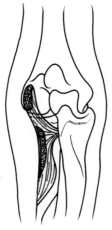

Position of the supinator

| | | | C5 | C6 | | | | | | M. biceps brachii |
| | | | C5 | C6 | C7 | | | | | M. supinator |

General comments

The basic movement is supination (lateral rotation) of the forearm. With a starting position of pronation the full range of movement is 180 degrees.

Grades 5, 4 and 3 are tested in sitting. Grades 2, 1 and 0 are tested in prone lying with the upper arm abducted and the forearm hanging over the edge of the plinth. The elbow is supported either by the examiner's hand or by a small pillow.

Fixation is necessary when testing grades 5 and 4, even if the muscles of the shoulder girdle are strong. When the muscles are weak, the greater part of the forearm must be supported when testing grade 3.

The supinator is situated very deep and can only be palpated if there is complete and simultaneous relaxation of the superficial extensors of the forearm.

The range of movement is limited by the ligaments, the interosseous membrane (distal part) and the pronators of the forearm.

Table 20.1

Prime mover	Origin	Insertion	Innervation
Biceps brachii	Long head: supraglenoid tubercle of scapula Short head: tip of coracoid process	Radial tuberosity of radius Bicipital aponeurosis into deep fascia over medial aspect of forearm and posterior border of ulna	Musculocutaneous nerve C5 C6
Supinator	Common extensor origin (lateral epicondyle of humerus)	Fibres run around neck of radius to attach to its anterior surface as far medially as anterior oblique line	Radial nerve (C5) C6 (C7)

Assisting muscles: Brachioradialis, from pronation to midposition
Stabilizers: Triceps and anconeus counteract flexion of biceps
Fixators: Triceps, anconeus and biceps fix the humeroulnar joint (flexion-extension)

Tests

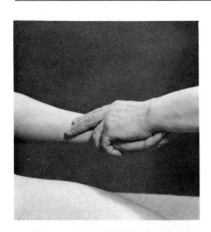
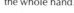

Grades 5, 4
Starting position: Sitting with the upper arm alongside the trunk, the elbow in 90-degree flexion and the forearm in pronation. The muscles of the wrist and fingers are relaxed.
Fixation: The upper arm just above the elbow.
Movement: Supination through the full range of movement.
Resistance: The examiner puts one hand into the hand of the patient with the index finger pointing towards the distal end of the ulna. Resistance is given with the whole hand.

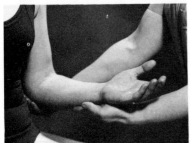

Grade 3
Starting position: Sitting with the upper arm alongside the trunk, the elbow in 90-degree flexion and the forearm in pronation. The muscles of the wrist and the fingers are relaxed.
Fixation: The upper arm just above the elbow. The examiner supports the forearm with the other hand.
Movement: Supination of the forearm through the full range of movement.

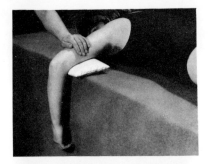

Grade 2
Starting position: Prone lying with the arm abducted to 90 degrees at the shoulder joint and the pronated forearm hanging over the edge of the plinth. The muscles of the wrist and the fingers are relaxed.
Fixation: The upper arm.
Movement: Supination through the full range of movement.

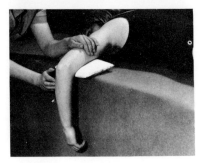

Grades 1, 0
Starting position: Prone lying with the upper arm abducted to 90 degrees at the shoulder joint and the elbow in 90-degree flexion. The forearm hangs over the edge of the plinth. The extensors of the wrist and the fingers are relaxed.
Fixation: Not necessary.
Movement: The supinator is palpated on the radial border of the proximal quarter of the forearm. The biceps brachii can be palpated close to its insertion in the fold of the elbow and along the course of its muscle fibres.

Possible errors

1. Flexion of the elbow at 90 degrees is not maintained.
2. The elbow does not remain in the same position and the upper arm is not fixed. The patient can initiate supination by flexion, adduction and lateral rotation of the shoulder joint. This particularly applies to grades 5, 4 and 3.
3. The muscles of the wrist and the fingers are not relaxed, and the extensors are active at the end of the movement.
4. With grades 5 and 4 the wrist is held incorrectly and may twist.

Shortening

With shortening the elbow is flexed and the forearm is supinated. Movements that demand pronation of the forearm are difficult to carry out.

99

21 The forearm:

Pronation

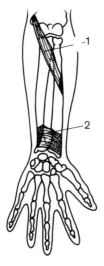

Pronation muscles of the forearm
(1) m. pronator teres, (2) m. pronator quadratus

| | | | C6 | C7 | | | | M. pronator teres |
| | | | C6 | C7 | C8 | T1 | | M. pronator quadratus |

General comments

The basic movement is pronation (medial rotation) of the forearm. The starting position is supination, and the full range of movement is 160 degrees.

Grades 5, 4 and 3 are tested in sitting. Grade 2 is tested in prone position. Grades 1 and 0 are tested in either prone or supine position. The fold of the elbow is supported by a small pillow. When testing for grade 3 function the forearm must always be supported. The pronator quadratus is located very deep and is difficult to palpate.

The range of movement is limited by the interosseous membrane (distal part), the medial collateral ligament of the radiocarpal joint and the posterior radiocarpal ligament.

Table 21.1

Prime mover	Origin	Insertion	Innervation
Pronator teres	Superficial head: common flexor origin Deep head: medial side of coronoid process of ulna	Middle of lateral surface of shaft of radius	Median nerve C6 (C7) Occasionally a few fibres from musculocutaneus nerve
Pronator quadratus	Lower quarter of anterior surface of ulna	Lower quarter of anterior surface of radius	Volar interosseous nerve medianus (C6) (C7) C8 T1

Assisting muscles: Flexor carpi radialis, palmaris longus, extensor carpi radialis longus
Stabilizers: Triceps brachii and anconeus counteract the flexion of pronator teres
Fixators: Triceps brachii, anconeus and biceps brachii fix the elbow

Tests

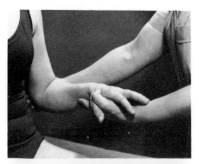

Grades 5, 4
Starting position: Sitting, with the upper arm alongside the trunk and the elbow in 90-degree flexion. The forearm is supinated. The muscles of the wrist and the fingers are relaxed.
Fixation: The examiner's palm and fingers are placed on the upper arm just above the elbow.
Movement: Pronation through the full range of movement.
Resistance: Just above the wrist on the anterior aspect of the forearm. The examiner grasps the patient's hand as if shaking hands and puts the index and middle fingers on the patient's wrist joint. Resistance is given by the whole hand, with particular pressure from the index finger on the styloid process of the radius.

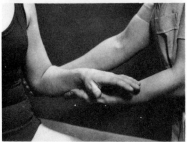

Grade 3
Starting position: Sitting with the upper arm alongside the trunk. The elbow is in 90-degree flexion, the forearm is supinated and the muscles of the wrist and the fingers are relaxed.
Fixation: The examiner places one hand on the upper arm just above the elbow and the other hand supports the forearm.
Movement: Pronation of the forearm through the full range of movement.

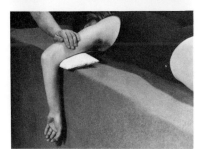

Grade 2
Starting position: Prone lying with the arm in 90-degree abduction at the shoulder joint, the elbow in 90-degree flexion and the forearm in supination and hanging over the edge of the plinth. The muscles of the wrist and the fingers are relaxed.
Fixation: The upper arm just above the elbow.
Movement: Pronation of the forearm through the full range of movement.

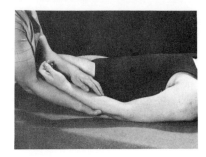

Grades 1, 0
Starting position: Supine lying with the arms beside the trunk and the elbows slightly flexed and in supination.
Movement: The pronator teres is palpated on the anterior aspect of the forearm just distal to the elbow and the pronator quadratus is palpated just above the wrist.

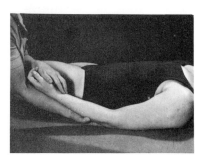

Possible errors

1. Necessary fixation of the upper arm is ignored. The patient can thus incorrectly initiate pronation of the forearm by abduction and medial rotation of the shoulder joint.
2. The elbow is not flexed to 90 degrees and does not remain in the same position.
3. The movement is finished by the flexors of the wrist and the fingers.

Shortening
If this occurs, the forearm is pronated and supination is made difficult.

22 The wrist joint:

Flexion with adduction (palmar flexion with ulnar deviation)

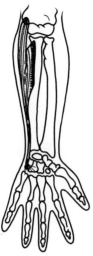

Position of the m. flexor carpi ulnaris

| | | | C7 | C8 | T1 | | | M. flexor carpi ulnaris |

General comments

The basic movement is flexion and adduction (ulnar deviation). The range of movement for flexion is 60 degrees or more, and for ulnar deviation is almost 60 degrees.

Flexion of the wrist is due to two-joint muscles, namely the flexor carpi radialis and the flexor carpi ulnaris, supported by the palmaris longus if present. By testing, the strength of one or the other can be well differentiated. Because both muscles originate from the humerus the starting position must be maintained carefully.

All grades are tested in sitting or supine position with the arm resting on the plinth. For grades 5, 4 and 3 the forearm is in supination, and for grades 2, 1 and 0 it is held between supination and the midposition. The fingers are relaxed during the test and at the end of the movement they are even slightly extended due to the tension of the extensors of the fingers.

Fixation of the forearm is necessary to ensure a correct starting position.

The range of movement is limited by the ligaments of the radial aspect of the wrist. In pathological conditions shortened extensors of the wrist and the fingers may decrease the range in the same way. This is shown by the increased extension of the fingers towards the end of the wrist flexion movement.

Table 22.1

Prime mover	Origin	Insertion	Innervation
Flexor carpi ulnaris	Humeral head: common flexor origin on the medial border of humerus Ulnar head: upper two thirds of posterior border of ulna olecranon	Pisiform bone, hamate bone and medial aspect of base of fifth metacarpal	Ulnar nerve (C7) C8 (T1)

Tests

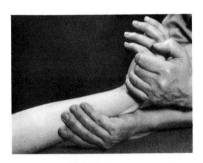

Grades 5, 4
Starting position: Sitting or supine lying with the arm resting on the plinth. The forearm is in supination with the dorsum on the plinth and the fingers completely relaxed.
Fixation: The distal third of the forearm, without pressing on the main muscle.
Movement: Simultaneous flexion and ulnar deviation at the wrist. The fingers are relaxed; however, towards the end of the movement they extend due to passive stretching of the extensors.
Resistance: With the palm against the direction of movement. The main pressure is against the hypothenar eminence.

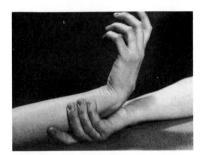

Grade 3
Starting position: Sitting or supine lying with the arm resting on the plinth. The forearm is in supination with the dorsum on the plinth and the fingers relaxed.
Fixation: The distal third of the forearm.
Movement: Flexion and ulnar deviation through the full range of movement.

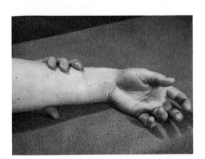

Grade 2
Starting position: Supine lying or sitting with the arm resting on the plinth, the forearm between supination and the midposition, the hand as an extension of the forearm and the fingers relaxed.
Fixation: The distal third of the forearm is grasped, leaving the wrist to move alone.
Movement: Flexion and ulnar deviation of the wrist joint. The ulnar border glides over the plinth while the fingers remain relaxed.

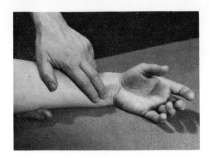

Grades 1, 0
Starting position: Supine lying or sitting with the forearm between supination and the midposition.
Movement: Muscle contraction can be palpated over the tendon proximal to its insertion, on the pisiform bone on its ulnar border and on the palmar aspect of the wrist.

Possible errors

Mistakes are rare if the tests are performed correctly.

1. The fingers are not relaxed throughout the movement.
2. There is often a tendency to perform substitution movements. This applies in particular to the little finger, which partly flexes at the metacarpophalangeal joint and partly extends at the interphalangeal joints. As proof of correct relaxation of the fingers there is some finger extension towards the end of the wrist movement.

Shortening

When this occurs, flexion and ulnar deviation, and limited extension and radial deviation are seen at the wrist joint.

23 The wrist joint:

Flexion with abduction (palmar flexion with radial deviation)

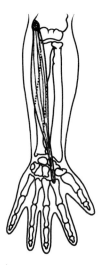

Position of m. flexor carpi radialis

| | | C6 | C7 | C8 | | | | | M. flexor carpi radialis |

General comments

The basic movement is flexion with abduction (radial deviation). The range of movement of flexion is 60 degrees and of radial deviation is up to 30 degrees.

All grades are examined in supine lying or in sitting with the arm resting on the plinth. Grades 5, 4 and 3 are tested from a starting position of slight flexion at the elbow joint with the forearm between midposition and pronation. In all grades the fingers must be completely relaxed.

Fixation of the forearm is necessary for all grades.

The range of movement is limited partly by the contact between the trapezium and the styloid processes of the radius and partly by the ulnar ligament of the wrist joint.

Table 23.1

Prime mover	Origin	Insertion	Innervation
Flexor carpi radialis	Common flexor origin on the medial epicondyle of humerus	Palmar surface of bases of second and third metacarpals	Median nerve C6 (C7) (C8)

Assisting muscles: Long flexors of the fingers and thumb

Tests

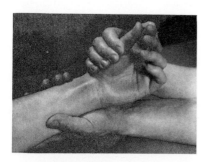

Grades 5, 4
Starting position: Supine lying or sitting. The arm rests on the plinth with a slight degree of flexion at the elbow joint. The forearm is between supination and the midposition. The fingers are completely relaxed.
Fixation: The examiner grasps the forearm with one hand to fix the posterior aspect of the distal third.
Movement: Simultaneous flexion and radial deviation at the wrist joint through the full range of movement.
Resistance: On the thenar eminence.

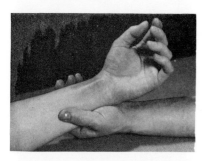

Grade 3
Starting position: Supine lying or sitting with the elbow slightly flexed and the forearm between supination and the midposition. The fingers are relaxed.
Fixation: The distal third of the forearm.
Movement: Flexion and radial deviation at the wrist joint.

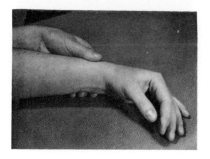

Grade 2
Starting position: Supine lying or sitting. The arm rests on the plinth with the elbow slightly flexed and the forearm between pronation and the midposition. The fingers are completely relaxed.
Fixation: The distal third of the forearm.
Movement: Flexion and radial deviation, the fingers sliding over the plinth.

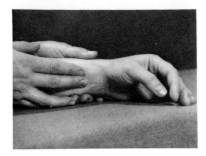

Grades 1, 0

Starting position: The forearm is between pronation and the midposition.

Movement: Increased tension can be palpated in the tendon of the flexor carpi radialis, on the lateral and anterior aspect of the distal part of the forearm and over the flexor retinaculum.

Possible errors

1. The correct starting position for the forearm and wrist is not observed.
2. The fingers, and in particular the thumb, are not completely relaxed during the whole movement.
3. There is an active attempt to flex the fingers during the test, which shows a tendency to substitution by the flexors of the fingers. The movement may also be assisted by activity of the flexor and the abductor of the thumb.
4. On palpation of the muscle contraction the tension of the other flexors that run adjacent is included. The radial pulse may be mistaken for a contraction.

Shortening

This causes slight flexion and radial deviation of the wrist joint, with a tendency towards pronation of the forearm.

24   The wrist joint:

Extension with adduction (dorsal flexion with ulnar deviation)

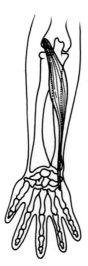

Position of m. extender carpi ulnaris

| | |C6 |C7 |C8 | | | | M. extensor carpi ulnaris

General comments

The basic movement is extension and adduction (ulnar deviation) of the wrist joint. The range of movement of extension is 70 degrees and of adduction is 60–70 degrees. Extension is carried out by two main groups of muscles. The result of their simultaneous contraction is pure extension of the wrist joint. When testing, the two muscle groups are discriminated by different starting positions and by a change in the direction of movement.

All grades are examined in sitting or supine positions. In grades 5, 4 and 3 the forearm is in pronation, while in grades 2, 1 and 0 the forearm is in a position between pronation and the midposition, with the hand as a prolongation of the forearm. The fingers must be relaxed throughout the test. Towards the end of the movement the fingers may be flexed passively by tension of the flexors. If there is a tendency for extension of the fingers during the test this shows attempted substitution by the common extensors of the fingers.

Fixation is necessary to keep the forearm in the correct position.

The range of movement is limited by the radial ligament of the wrist joint.

Table 24.1

Prime mover	Origin	Insertion	Innervation
Extensor carpi ulnaris	Common extensor origin on the lateral epicondyle of the humerus; by an aponeurotic attachment to posterior border of ulna	Ulnar side of base of fifth metacarpal	Radial nerve (C6) C7 (C8)

Tests

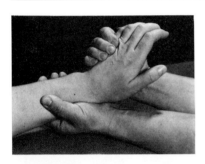

Grades 5, 4
Starting position: Supine lying or sitting. The arm rests on the plinth with the forearm in pronation and the hand as an extension of the forearm. The fingers are relaxed.
Fixation: Anterior aspect of the distal third of the forearm. The posterior aspect remains free and the wrist joint must not be restricted.
Movement: Simultaneous extension and ulnar deviation of the wrist joint with the full range of movement.
Resistance: With the examiner's palm on the dorsum of the hand. Pressure is mainly directed towards the head of the fifth metacarpal.

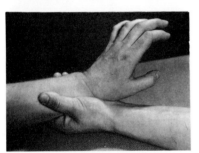

Grade 3
Starting position: Supine lying or sitting. The arm rests on the plinth and the forearm is in pronation with the hand as an extension of the forearm. The fingers are relaxed.
Fixation: Distal third of the forearm (anterior aspect).
Movement: Extension with ulnar deviation.

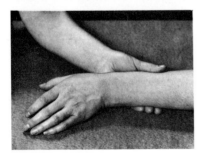

Grade 2
Starting position: Supine lying or sitting. The forearm is in a position between pronation and the midposition with the hand as an extension of the forearm. The fingers are relaxed.
Fixation: The examiner's whole hand grips the distal third of the forearm.
Movement: Extension with ulnar deviation. The ulnar border of the hand slides over the support through the full range of movement. The fingers remain at rest, or possibly tend to flex.

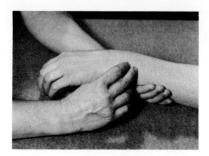

Grades 1, 0
Starting position: Supine lying or sitting.
Movement: The tension in the tendon of the extensor carpi ulnaris can be palpated just distal to the styloid process of the ulna, on the posterior aspect. The wrist joint must be flexed maximally to bring the extensors of the wrist into an initial stretch.

Possible errors

1. Fixation is often ignored.
2. The fingers do not remain relaxed throughout the movement. They must not extend, but they are pulled into flexion by the passively stretched flexor muscles towards the end of the test. If there is a simultaneous tendency to extend the fingers, this is due to substitution by the extensor digitorum.

Shortening

With shortening the wrist joint is slightly extended and in marked ulnar deviation.

25 The wrist joint:

Extension with abduction (dorsal flexion with radial deviation)

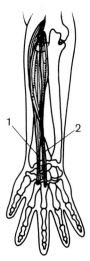

Position of muscles allowing wrist extension with abduction
(1) m. extensor carpi radialis longus, (2) m. extensor carpi radialis brevis

		C5	C6	C7	C8				M. extensor carpi radialis longus
		C5	C6	C7	C8				M. extensor carpi radialis brevis

General comments

The basic movement is extension and abduction (radial deviation) at the wrist joint. The range of movement for extension is 70–80 degrees and for radial deviation is 20–30 degrees.

In grades 5, 4, 3, 1 and 0 the forearm is between pronation and the midposition. In grade 2 the forearm is between supination and the midposition. The hand is held as an extension of the forearm. During the complete movement the fingers are fully relaxed. They do not extend but rather show a tendency to flex due to passive stretching of the flexors towards the end of the test.

Fixation is necessary to keep the forearm still and in the correct position.

The range of movement is limited by the contact between the trapezium and the styloid process of the radius, and also by the palmar radiocarpal ligament and the medial collateral ligament of the wrist joint.

Table 25.1

Prime mover	Origin	Insertion	Innervation
Extensor carpi radialis longus	Lower third of lateral supracondylar ridge of humerus	Dorsal surface of base of second metacarpal	Radial nerve (C5) C6 C7 (C8)
Extensor carpi radialis brevis	Common extensor origin on the lateral epicondyle of humerus	Posterior aspect of base of third metacarpal	Radial nerve (c5) C6 C7 (C8)

Assisting muscles: Abductor pollicis longus, extensor pollicis longus, extensor pollicis brevis

Tests

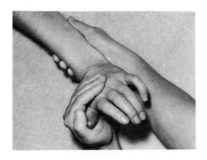

Grades 5, 4
Starting position: Supine lying or sitting. The arm rests on the plinth with the forearm pronated and the hand as an extension of the forearm. The fingers are slightly flexed.
Fixation: The forearm is supported on its anterior aspect. Movement of the wrist joint must not be restricted.
Movement: Simultaneous extension and radial deviation with the full range of movement. The fingers remain relaxed or show some tendency to flexion.
Resistance: With the examiner's whole palm on the dorsum of the hand. The main resistance is given over the metacarpophalangeal joint of the index finger. The direction of the resistance is against flexion and ulnar deviation.

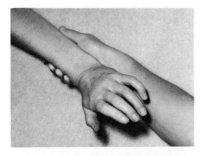

Grade 3
Starting position: Supine lying or sitting with the arm resting on the plinth the forearm pronated and the hand as an extension of the forearm. The fingers are relaxed.
Fixation: The examiner's palm and fingers on the anterior aspect of the forearm.
Movement: Extension and radial deviation at the wrist.

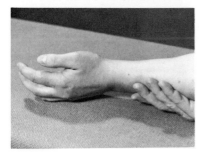

Grade 2
Starting position: Supine lying or sitting. The arm rests on the plinth with the forearm between supination and the midposition and the hand as an extension of the forearm. The ulnar border is supported and the fingers are relaxed throughout the movement.
Movement: Extension and radial deviation. During the movement the ulnar border slides over the support.

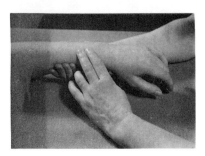

Grades 1, 0

Movement: The tendons of the extensor carpi radialis longus and the extensor carpi radialis brevis can be palpated just proximal to the second metacarpal on the dorsum of the hand, deep to the posterior ligament of the wrist joint. The wrist is slightly flexed in order to stretch the extensors.

Possible errors

1. The fingers do not remain relaxed during the movement. They may be slightly flexed by passive stretching of the flexors. A tendency towards active extension is due to substitution by the common extensor of the fingers.

Other mistakes are rare if the correct starting position is maintained.

Shortening

This causes extension and radial deviation of the wrist joint. There is also a limited range of flexion and ulnar deviation.

26 The metacarpophalangeal joints of the fingers:

Flexion

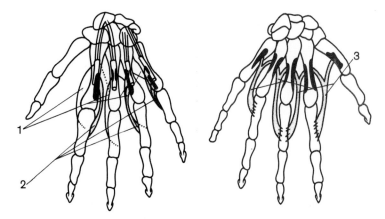

Flexion muscles of the metacarpophalangeal finger joints
(1) mm. lumbricales, (2) mm. interossei palmares, (3) mm. interossei dorsales

			C7	C8	T1				Mm. lumbricales I, II
			C7	**C8**	**T1**				Mm. lumbricales III, IV
				C8	T1				Mm. interossei dorsales
				C8	T1				Mm. interossei palmares

General comments

The basic movement is flexion at the metacarpophalangeal joints with the interphalangeal joints extended. The range of movement is 90 degrees.

All tests are carried out in supine lying or sitting. The forearm rests on the examination plinth and is in supination for grades 5, 4, 3, 1 and 0 and in the midposition for grade 2.

Fixation of the hand is necessary for all grades. The hand must remain as an extension of the forearm during the complete movement.

The lumbricales are mainly flexors of the metacarpophalangeal joints but they also assist in extension of the interphalangeal joints by their insertion into the posterior aponeurosis of the fingers.

The range of movement is mainly limited by the structures of the joints.

115

Table 26.1

Prime mover	Origin	Insertion	Innervation
Lumbricales	In the palm from radial side of each of four tendons of flexor digitorum profundus	Radial side of dorsal expansion of same finger (proximal phalanx)	Lumbricales manus laterales: median nerve C7 C8 T1 Lumbricales manus mediales: ulnar nerve (C7) C8 T1
Interossei dorsales from radial side they are four	Two heads from adjacent sides of metacarpals	Corresponding proximal phalanx and extensor expansion: 1 and 2 on radial side of index and middle fingers, 3 and 4 on ulnar side of middle and ring fingers (middle finger has two dorsal interossei)	Ulnar nerve C8 (T1)
Interossei palmares they are three	Shafts of metacarpals 2, 4 and 5 (ulnar side of second metacarpal, radial side of fourth and fifth metacarpals)	Base of corresponding proximal phalanx and extensor expansion (middle finger has no interosseus palmaris)	Ulnar nerve C8 (T1)

Assisting muscles: Flexor digitorum profundus, flexor digiti minimi brevis, flexor digitorum superficialis

Tests

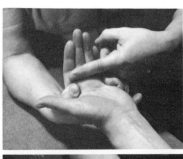

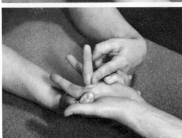

Grades 4, 5
Starting position: Supine lying or sitting. The elbow is slightly flexed, the forearm is in supination and relaxed on the plinth and the fingers are extended.
Fixation: The heads of the metacarpals.
Movement: Flexion at metacarpophalangeal joints 1–4 simultaneously or, better, individually. The interphalangeal joints remain extended.
Resistance: On the palmar aspect of the proximal phalanges, that is on fingers 2–5 simultaneously or individually.

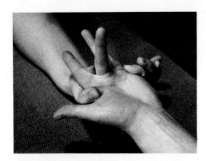

Grade 3

Starting position: Supine lying or sitting. The forearm rests in supination on the plinth. The fingers are in extension at all their joints.

Fixation: Heads of the metacarpals.

Movement: Flexion at the metacarpophalangeal joints of fingers 2–5, either simultaneously or, better, individually.

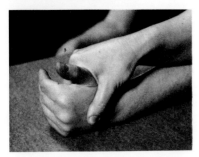

Grade 2

Starting position: Supine lying or sitting with the forearm in the midposition resting on the plinth and the fingers extended.

Fixation: Metacarpals.

Movement: Flexion at the metacarpophalangeal joints with the exception of the thumb. The interphalangeal joints remain extended.

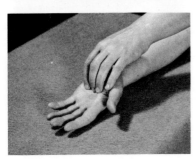

Grades 1, 0

Movement: Contraction of the lumbricales can be palpated on the palm. The fingers are extended at the interphalangeal joints with the hand as an extension of the forearm.

Possible errors

1. Fixation of the metacarpals is ignored.
2. The hand is not held as an extension of the forearm or the fingers are not extended at the interphalangeal joints.
3. Movement takes place at the metacarpophalangeal joints alone.
4. Resistance is not carefully given to the proximal phalanges and it affects the middle or distal phalanges.

Shortening

Flexion at the metacarpophalangeal and extended interphalangeal joints results from shortening. If there is hyperextension of the metacarpophalangeal joints, flexion of the interphalangeal joints is impossible. Conversely, extension of the metacarpophalangeal joints is impossible if there is flexion of the interphalangeal joints.

117

27 The metacarpophalangeal joints of the fingers:

Extension

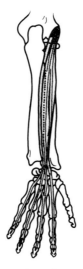

Position of m. extensor digitorum

			C5	C6	C7			M. extensor digitorum
				C6	C7	C8		M. extensor indicis
					C7	C8		M. extensor digiti minimi

General comments

The basic movement is extension at the metacarpophalangeal joints from a starting position of maximal flexion. The range of movement is 100 degrees. For grades 5, 4, 3, 1 and 0 the arm is in pronation, and for grade 2 it is in the midposition.

In all grades fixation is absolutely necessary.

Resistance is best given to each finger individually. During movement the fingers are relaxed and slightly flexed at the interphalangeal joints.

The range of movement is limited by the joint capsule, on the palmar aspect by the ligaments of the palm and in pathological cases by the flexor muscles.

Table 27.1

Prime mover	Origin	Insertion	Innervation
Extensor digitorum	Common extensor origin on the lateral epicondyle of humerus	By four tendons to posterior aspect of base of middle and distal phalanges	Radial nerve (C5) C6 (C7)
Extensor indicis	Third quarter of posterior surface of ulna and adjacent interosseus membrane distal to extensor pollicis longus	Unites with index finger tendon of extensor digitorum	Radial nerve (C6) C7 (C8)
Extensor digiti minimi	Common extensor origin	Unites with little finger tendon of extensor digitorum	Radial nerve C7 (C8)

Stabilizers: Flexor digitorum superficialis keeps the interphalangeal joints flexed

Tests

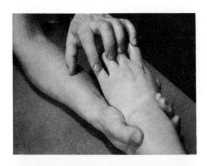

Grades 5, 4
Starting position: Supine lying or sitting with the elbow slightly flexed, the forearm supported in pronation on the plinth and the hand as an extension of the forearm. The patient's hand is supported by the examiner's palm. The fingers are slightly flexed at the interphalangeal joints and fully flexed at the metacarpophalangeal joints.
Fixation: The wrist and palm are grasped from the anterior aspect and the patient's hand is held as an extension of the forearm.
Movement: Extension at the metacarpophalangeal joints through the full range of movement.
Resistance: On the posterior aspect of the metacarpophalangeal joints of fingers 2–5.

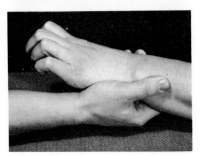

Grade 3
Starting position: Supine lying or sitting with the forearm pronated, the elbow slightly flexed and the hand as an extension of the forearm. The fingers are slightly flexed at the interphalangeal joints and fully flexed at the metacarpophalangeal joints.
Fixation: Wrist joint and hand.
Movement: Extension at the metacarpophalangeal joints through the full range of movement.

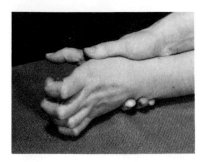

Grade 2
Starting position: Supine lying or sitting with the elbow slightly flexed, the forearm resting on the ulnar border on the plinth and the hand as an extension of the forearm. The fingers are slightly flexed at the interphalangeal joints and fully flexed at the metacarpophalangeal joints.
Fixation: The wrist and hand are firmly grasped by the examiner's palm.
Movement: Extension at the metacarpophalangeal joints through the full range of movement.

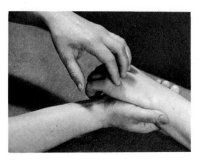

Grades 1, 0
Starting position: Supine lying or sitting with the forearm resting on the plinth.
Movement: The tendon of the extensor digitorum can be palpated on the posterior aspect over the metacarpals.

Possible errors

1. Extension at the interphalangeal joints is often carried out by the lumbricales and wrongly characterized as extension by the long extensor. In this way there may be mistaken diagnosis of a peripheral nerve lesion of the radial or ulnar nerve.
2. If there is inadequate fixation of the wrist joint the activity of the wrist extensors may imitate the strength of the finger extensors.

Shortening

When this is present the extensors of the fingers are pulled into hyperextension during flexion of the wrist joint.

28 The metacarpophalangeal joints of the fingers:

Adduction

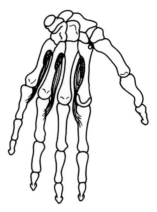

Position of m. interossei palmares

| | | **C8** | **T1** | | | | Mm. interossei palmares |

General comments

The basic movement is adduction of the fingers from a starting position of abduction. It is carried out by the interossei palmares. There are three interossei, serving the second, fourth and fifth fingers.

For grade 3 two starting positions are used to test all the muscles. In grades 5 and 4 resistance is given on each individual finger.

The range of movement is limited by the contact between the fingers.

Table 28.1

Prime mover	Origin	Insertion	Innervation
Interossei palmares	Shafts of metacarpals 2, 4 and 5 (ulnar side of second metacarpal, radial side of fourth and fifth)	Base of corresponding proximal phalanx and extensor expansion (middle finger *has no* interosseus palmaris)	Ulnar nerve C8–T1

Assisting muscles: Extensor indicis (for the index finger)

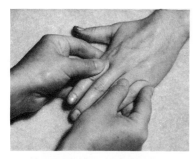

Grades 5, 4
Starting position: Supine lying or sitting. The forearm and hand rest on the plinth on the anterior aspect, and the abducted fingers are supported.
Fixation: The fingers are supported as well as given resistance from underneath.
Movement: From maximal abduction fingers 2, 4 and 5 are adducted.
Resistance: On the palmar and dorsal aspects of the proximal phalanx.

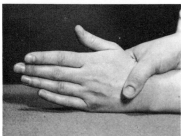

Grade 3
Starting position: Supine lying or sitting with the forearm on the plinth on the ulnar border for testing fingers 4 and 5 and on the radial border for testing finger 2.
Fixation: The wrist joint.
Movement: Adduction of the individual fingers according to the starting position (towards the middle finger).

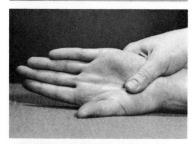

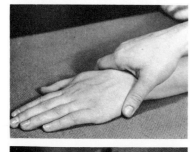

Grade 2
Starting position: Supine lying or sitting. The forearm, hand and fingers rest on their anterior aspects on the plinth. The fingers are abducted.
Fixation: Not necessary.
Movement: Adduction of fingers 2, 4 and 5. The middle finger remains at rest.

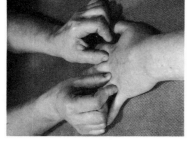

Grades 1, 0
Starting position: The forearm, hand and fingers rest in pronation on the plinth. The fingers are slightly abducted.
Movement: Contraction is palpated over the proximal phalanx of fingers 2, 4 and 5. It is enough for a muscle pull to be felt in the direction of movement.

Posible errors

Errors are rare.

Shortening

This causes flexion and adduction of the metacarpophalangeal joints and extension of the interphalangeal joints. Flexion at the interphalangeal joints is impossible with hyperextended meta-carpophalangeal joints and conversely extension at the meta-carpophalangeal joints is impossible with flexed interphalangeal joints.

29 The metacarpophalangeal joints of the fingers:

Abduction

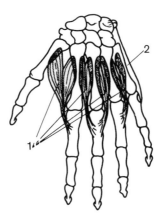

Abduction muscles of the metacarpophalangeal finger joints
(1) mm. interossei dorsales, (2) m. abductor digiti minimi

| | | | C8 | T1 | | | | Mm. interossei dorsales |
| | | C7 | C8 | T1 | | | | M. abductor digiti minimi |

General comments

The basic movement is abduction of the extended finger with a range of movement of 20–25 degrees.

In grades 5 and 4 each finger is tested individually. In grade 3 two starting positions are used to enable testing of all the fingers.

Resistance is given against the proximal phalanx to exclude influence from the other finger joints and lessen the assistance of other muscles. There are four interossei dorsales manus, two of which insert on the middle finger.

The range of movement is limited mainly by the structures of the joints.

Table 29.1

Prime mover	Origin	Insertion	Innervation
Interossei dorsales manus	Two heads from adjacent sides of metacarpals	Base of corresponding proximal phalanx and extension expansion (1 and 2 on the radial side of the index and middle fingers, 3 and 4 on the ulnar side of the middle and ring fingers)	Ulnar nerve C8 (T1)
Abductor digiti minimi manus	Pisiform bone, flexor retinaculum	Ulnar side of base of proximal phalanx of little finger	Ulnar nerve (C7) C8 T1

Tests

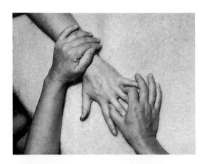

Grades 5, 4
Starting position: Supine lying or sitting. The forearm, the hand and the fingers (in adduction) rest on the palmar aspect on the table.
Fixation: The wrist and the distal third of the forearm are gently pressed against the support.
Movement: Abduction through the full range of movement.
Resistance: On each individual finger on the radial or ulnar aspect of the proximal phalanx. On the middle finger resistance is given on both the ulnar and the radial side.

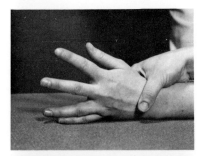

Grade 3
Starting position: Supine lying or sitting. The forearm rests on the plinth, first on the ulnar aspect and then on the radial aspect.
Fixation: The wrist and the forearm.
Movement: Abduction of the fingers through the full range of movement according to the starting position. First the index and middle fingers are examined, that is the first and second interosseus dorsalis manus. Then the middle, ring and little fingers are examined, that is the third and fourth interosseus dorsalis manus and the abductor digiti minimi. In this way the middle finger is tested twice.

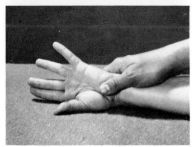

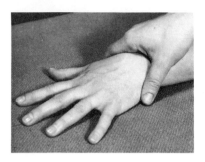

Grade 2
Starting position: Supine lying or sitting. The forearm, the hand and the fingers (in adduction) rest on the palmar aspect on the plinth.
Fixation: The wrist.
Movement: Abduction of the fingers through the full range of movement. The middle finger is tested in both ulnar and radial directions.

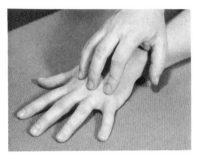

Grades 1, 0
Starting position: The forearm, the hand and the fingers rest relaxed and in pronation on the plinth.
Movement: The contractions of the individual muscles are palpated one by one between the metacarpal heads. However, it is safer to observe the muscle pull in the direction of movement.

Possible errors

Mistakes are rare.

Shortening

If this occurs then the fingers are in extension. When the metacarpophalangeal joints are in maximal flexion, flexion of the interphalangeal joints is impossible. Conversely flexion of the metacarpophalangeal joints is impossible when the interphalangeal joints are flexed.

30 The proximal interphalangeal joints of the fingers:

Flexion

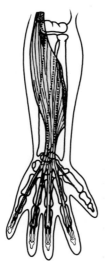

Position of m. flexor digitorum superficialis

| | | C7 | C8 | T1 | | | M. flexor digitorum superficialis

General comments

The basic movement is flexion of the proximal interphalangeal joints with the metacarpophalangeal joints extended. The range of movement is about 100 degrees.

All tests are carried out lying or sitting. The forearm rests in supination on the plinth. There is no distinction between grades 3 and 2 because of the small weight of the phalanges. The fingers are tested individually.

Fixation is important. The proximal phalanx is grasped on either side by the thumb and the middle finger, and the index finger supports the metacarpal head. In this way the metacarpophalangeal joint is held in slight extension (*Picture a*).

The range of movement is limited by the articulating surfaces of the joint.

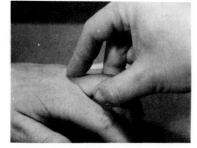

(a)

Table 30.1

Prime mover	Origin	Insertion	Innervation
Flexor digitorum superficialis	Humeroulnar head: common flexor origin, ulnar collateral ligament of elbow joint, tubercle on coronoid process Radial head: anterior oblique line on the radius	Four tendons passing to each finger are attached to sides of middle phalanx	Median nerve C7 C8 T1 Occasionally also ulnar nerve

Tests

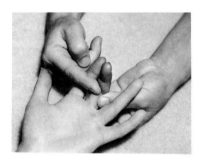

Grades 5, 4
Starting position: Supine lying or sitting with the elbow slightly flexed. The forearm is in supination with the hand resting as an extension of the forearm and the fingers are extended.
Fixation: The proximal phalanx of the finger is held so that the metacarpophalangeal joint remains in hyperextension throughout the test.
Movement: Flexion of the proximal interphalangeal joint through the full range of movement.
Resistance: On the anterior aspect of the middle phalanx.

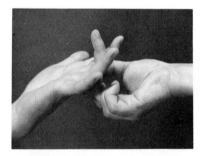

Grades 3, 2
Starting position, fixation and movement: As for grades 5 and 4, without resistance.

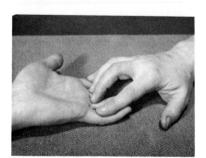

Grades 1, 0
Starting position: Supine lying or sitting with the elbow slightly flexed and the forearm in supination.
Movement: The tendon can be palpated on the anterior aspect of the proximal phalanx.

Possible errors

1. The hand is not held as an extension of the forearm.
2. Correct flexion and the necessary hyperextension of the metacarpophalangeal joint are not carried out.
3. The proximal interphalangeal joint does not remain in extension.

Shortening

If shortening occurs then with an·extended wrist joint there is flexion of the metacarpophalangeal and proximal interphalangeal joints.

31 The distal interphalangeal joints of the fingers:

Flexion

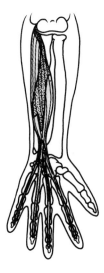

Position of m. flexor digitorum profundus

			C7	C8	T1				M. flexor digitorum profundus II
			C7	C8	T1				M. flexor digitorum profundus III, IV, V

General comments

The basic movement is flexion of the distal interphalangeal joints with the other finger joints in extension. The range of movement is about 80 degrees.

All grades are examined with the forearm in supination. There is no distinction between grades 3 and 2 due to the low weight of the fingers. Each finger is tested individually. Simultaneous examination of all the fingers is not exact and is insufficient for assessment.

Fixation is the same as for the proximal interphalangeal joints, with the difference that the proximal interphalangeal joint is held in extension (*Picture a*).

The range of movement is limited by the articulating surfaces.

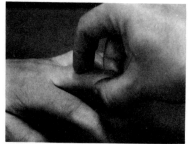

(a)

Table 31.1

Prime mover	Origin	Insertion	Innervation
Flexor digitorum profundus	Anterior and medial surfaces and posterior border of upper three quarters of ulna and adjacent interosseous membrane	Each of the four tendons passes to base of distal phalanx of finger concerned	Medial part of ulnar nerve, lateral part of anterior interosseus nerve

Tests

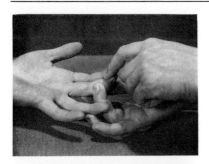

Grades 5, 4
Starting position: Supine lying or sitting. The elbow is slightly flexed and the forearm is in supination with the hand as an extension of the forearm and the fingers are extended.
Fixation: The middle phalanx from each side.
Movement: Flexion of the distal interphalangeal joint through the full range of movement.
Resistance: On the anterior aspect of the distal phalanx of the finger.

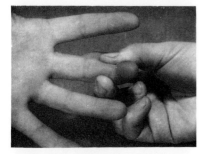

Grades 3–2
Starting position: The forearm is in supination with the hand held as an extension of the forearm and the fingers extended.
Fixation: The middle phalanx.
Movement: Flexion of the distal interphalangeal joint.

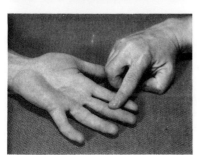

Grades 1, 0
Starting position: Supine lying or sitting with the elbow slightly flexed, the forearm in supination and the fingers extended.
Movement: The tendon of the flexor digitorum profundus can be palpated on the palmar aspect of the middle phalanx of the tested finger.

Possible errors

1. The wrist joint is not extended.
2. There is fixation of the middle phalanx alone. The fingers must be fixed from either side so that there is no pressure on the tendon during the movement.
3. The other finger joints do not remain extended during the entire movement.

Shortening

This causes flexion of all the finger joints.

32 The carpometacarpal (saddle) joint of the thumb:

Adduction

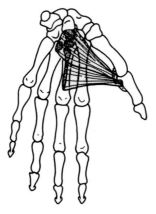

Position of m. adductor pollicis

| | | | C7 | C8 | T1 | | | M. adductor pollicis |

General comments

The basic movement is adduction of the thumb from a starting position of abduction. The range of movement is 50 degrees.

In grades 5, 4, 2, 1 and 0 the forearm is pronated. In grade 3 it rests on the radial border. The adduction of the thumb is tested in such a way that the thumb remains in the plane of the palm during the entire movement. Movement at 90 degrees to the palm is due not to activity of the adductor pollicis but mainly to activity of the interossei dorsales manus (namely palmar adduction).

The range of movement is limited by approximation of the thumb and the second metacarpal.

Table 32.1

Prime mover	Origin	Insertion	Innervation
Adductor pollicis	Transverse head: palmar surface of third shaft of metacarpal Oblique head: palmar surface of bases of second and third metacarpals and adjacent carpal bones	By a small tendon into radial side of base of proximal phalanx Into ulnar side of base of proximal phalanx of thumb	Deep branch of ulnar nerve (C7) C8 (T1)

Assisting muscles: Flexor pollicis brevis, flexor pollicis longus, opponens, extensor pollicis longus, interossei dorsales manus

Tests

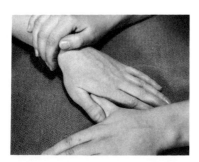

Grades 5, 4
Starting position: Supine lying or sitting. The forearm rests in pronation on the plinth with the hand as an extension of the forearm. The fingers are extended and the thumb is abducted.
Fixation: The wrist.
Movement: Adduction of the thumb in the plane of the palm through the full range of movement.
Resistance: Against the ulnar and palmar aspects of the thumb with the main pressure on the first metacarpal.

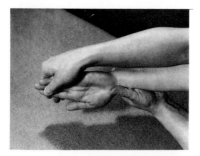

Grade 3
Starting position: Supine lying or sitting with the radial border of the forearm turned towards the plinth and the thumb abducted.
Fixation: The forearm is supported and the fingers are gripped.
Movement: Adduction of the thumb in the plane of the palm.

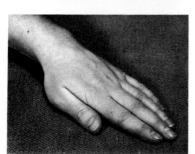

Grade 2
Starting position: Supine lying or sitting. The pronated forearm, the hand and the fingers rest on the plinth. The thumb is abducted.
Fixation: Not necessary.
Movement: Adduction of the thumb in the plane of the palm through the full range of movement.

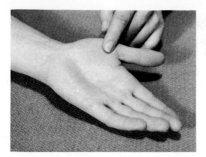

Grades 1, 0
Movement: A very weak contraction can be palpated between the first and second metacarpals at the insertion of the adductor pollicis on the palmar aspect.

Possible errors

1. The movement does not take place in the plane of the palm.
2. The thumb does not remain extended at the metacarpophalangeal and interphalangeal joints.

Shortening

With shortening the thumb is in adduction. Abduction through the full range of movement is impossible.

33   The carpometacarpal (saddle) joint of the thumb:

Abduction

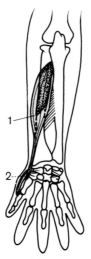

Abduction muscle of the carpometacarpal joint of the thumb
(1) m. abductor pollicis longus, (2) m. abductor pollicis brevis

		C6	C7	C8				M. abductor pollicis longus
		C6	C7	C8	T1			M. abductor pollicis brevis

General comments

The basic movement is abduction of the thumb through a range of movement of 60–70 degrees.

In grades 5, 4, 2, 1 and 0 the forearm is pronated on the plinth. In grade 3 it is midway between pronation and supination. The hand must remain held as an extension of the forearm during the entire movement.

Abduction of the thumb is carried out by two muscles, namely the abductor pollicis brevis and the abductor pollicis longus. A sideways movement in the plane of the palm is considered to be pure abduction and is carried out by the abductor pollicis longus assisted by the extensor pollicis brevis. The abductor pollicis brevis carries out movement at 90 degrees to the palm, that is palmar abduction. During this other muscles are active, including the abductor pollicis longus (which gives off a few muscle fibres to the abductor pollicis brevis), the flexor pollicis brevis and possibly also the opponens pollicis. However, palmar abduction is fairly complicated and without special practice even a healthy person is unable to perform it correctly. Because of this, only pure abduction is generally assessed and the abductor pollicis brevis is examined in an empirical fashion.

The range of movement is limited by approximation of the soft tissue of the thumb and the index finger.

Table 33.1

Prime mover	Origin	Insertion	Innervation
Abductor pollicis longus	Posterior surface of ulna below attachment of anconeus, second quarter of posterior surface of radius and intervening interosseous membrane	Radial side of base of first metacarpal	Radial nerve (C6) C7 (C8)
Abductor pollicis brevis	Tubercle of scaphoid and adjacent flexor retinaculum	Radial side of the base of the thumb	

Tests

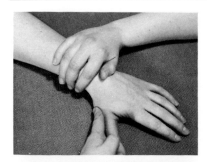

Grades 5, 4
Starting position: Supine lying or sitting with the forearm resting in pronation on the plinth, the hand as an extension of the forearm, the thumb adducted, and the fingers relaxed.
Fixation: The wrist.
Movement: Abduction of the thumb in the plane of the palm through the full range of movement.
Resistance: On the radial aspect of the first metacarpal.

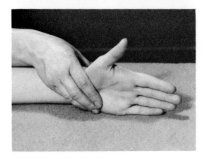

Grade 3
Starting position: Supine lying or sitting with the forearm in the midposition and the ulnar border resting on the plinth. The hand is held as an extension of the forearm, the thumb is adducted and the fingers are relaxed.
Fixation: The wrist joint.
Movement: Abduction of the thumb in the plane of the palm.

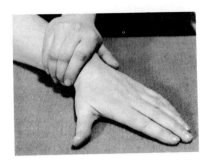

Grade 2
Starting position: The forearm pronated on the plinth with the hand as an extension of the forearm and the thumb adducted.
Fixation: The wrist joint.
Movement: Abduction of the thumb through the full range of movement.

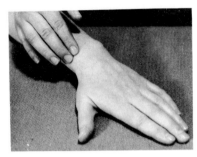

Grades 1, 0
Movement: The tendon of the abductor pollicis longus can be palpated over the styloid process of the radius and on the palmar edge of the anatomical snuffbox. The abductor pollicis brevis can be palpated laterally at the base of the thenar eminence.

Possible errors

1. The correct position of the forearm and hand is ignored.
2. The movement is not always in the plane of the palm.
3. The fixation of the hand is ignored and simultaneous movement at the wrist joint is allowed.

Shortening

This causes abduction of the thumb and shortening of the abductor pollicis longus. There is a slight radial deviation of the wrist.

34 The thumb and little finger:

Opposition

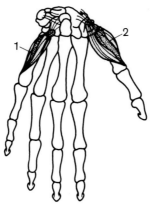

Opposition muscles of the thumb and little finger
(1) m. opponens digiti minimi, (2) m. opponens pollicis

			C6	C7	C8	T1				M. opponens pollicis
				C7	C8	T1				M. opponens digiti minimi

General comments

The basic movement is opposition of the thumb and little finger.
This is a complicated manoeuvre initiated by palmar abduction
at the saddle joint of the thumb, followed by ulnar adduction
which proceeds to the final position with slight flexion and
rotation at the metacarpophalangeal joint. Many muscles are
activated during the movement, including in the initial stage the
abductor muscles together with the flexor pollicis brevis and the
adductor pollicis. The opponens pollicis is only active as a prime
mover during actual opposition. The range of movement is about
60 degrees. The movement takes place at the saddle joint of the
thumb.

In opposition of the fifth finger, apart from the opponens digiti
minimi, the fourth lumbricalis manus, the abductor digiti minimi
manus and the flexor digiti minimi brevis are active. The main
actions of the opponens digiti minimi are rotation and
opposition. Movement is initiated at the fifth carpometacarpal
joint, where there is later flexion.

Grades 3 and 2 are not differentiated. During assessment of a
peripheral nerve lesion it must be noted that the opponens
pollicis is innervated by the median nerve whereas the opponens
digiti minimi is innervated by the ulnar nerve.

The range of movement is tested until there is contact between
the thumb and the little finger.

139

Table 34.1

Prime mover	Origin	Insertion	Innervation
Opponens pollicis	Ridge of trapezium and adjacent flexor retinaculum	Whole length of radial margin of first metacarpal	Median nerve (C6) (C7) (C8) (T1)
Opponens digiti minimi	Hook of hamate and adjacent flexor retinaculum	Whole length of ulnar margin of fifth metacarpal	Ulnar nerve (C7) C8 T1

Assisting muscles: Adductor pollicis, abductor pollicis brevis, abductor pollicis longus, flexor pollicis brevis, flexor pollicis longus

Stabilizers: In the second stage of the movement the flexor pollicis longus is prevented from causing flexion and radial deviation of the wrist by the action of the extensors. The extensor of the thumb limits the flexor pollicis brevis

Fixators: All the muscles of the thenar eminence affect each other

Tests

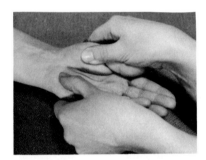

Grades 5, 4
Starting position: Supine lying or sitting. The forearm rests in supination on the table with the hand as an extension of the forearm and the fingers extended.
Fixation: Not necessary.
Movement: Opposition of the thumb and the little finger, with rotation stressed at the latter.
Resistance: On the palmar aspect of the first and fifth metacarpal heads.

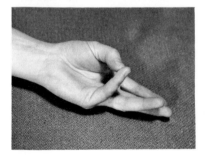

Grades 3−2
Starting position, fixation and movement: The same as grades 5 and 4, without resistance.

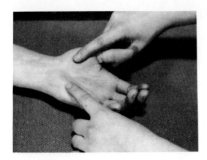

Grades 1, 0

Movement: The opponens pollicis can be palpated on the anterior and radial aspects of the first metacarpal. The opponens digiti minimi is difficult to palpate on the hypothenar eminence, and because of its deep localization its assessment is often unreliable.

Possible errors

1. The correct sequence of movement with palmar abduction of the thumb (which constitutes the main component of opposition) is not observed. Adduction and flexion of the thumb alone may be taken for opposition.
2. Resistance is not given correctly, that is mainly against opposition and not only against abduction, adduction and flexion.

Shortening

This is rare and is only manifested by slight rotation and opposition of the thumb or the little finger.

35 The metacarpophalangeal joint of the thumb:

Flexion

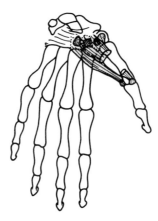

Position of m. flexor pollicis brevis, c. superficiale, c. profundum

| | | | C6 | C7 | C8 | T1 | | | | M. flexor pollicis brevis

General comments

The basic movement is flexion of the metacarpophalangeal joint of the thumb through a range of movement of 80–90 degrees. There are great variations in the mobility of the joint. During the test the forearm rests in supination on the examination plinth.

Fixation of the first metacarpal is necessary because flexion of the saddle joint of the thumb impairs the prospects of the movement, in particular at the end of the test.

Grades 3 and 2 are not differentiated.

The range of movement is limited by the structure of the joint.

Table 35.1

Prime mover	Origin	Insertion	Innervation
Flexor pollicis brevis	Ridge of trapezium and adjacent flexor retinaculum	Radial side of base of proximal phalanx of thumb	Median nerve C6,C7

Assisting muscles: Abductor pollicis brevis, adductor pollicis, flexor pollicis longus

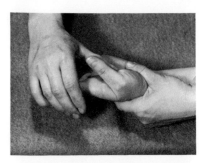

Grades 5, 4 ·
Starting position: Supine lying or sitting. The forearm is in supination on the plinth with the thumb extended and abducted and the fingers relaxed.
Fixation: The first metacarpal is fixed in the starting position without any pressure on the thenar eminence.
Resistance: The examiner presses one finger against the anterior aspect of the proximal phalanx of the thumb.

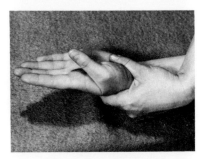

Grades 3–2
Starting position, fixation and movement: As for grades 5 and 4 with no resistance.

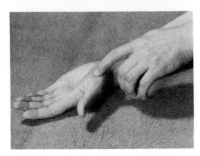

Grades 1, 0
Starting position: The forearm rests in supination on the plinth.
Fixation: The first metacarpal.
Movement: The flexor pollicis brevis can be palpated on the anterior aspect of the first metacarpal.

Possible errors

1. The first metacarpal is not firmly fixed.
2. There is flexion of the interphalangeal joint of the thumb.

36 The metacarpophalangeal joint of the thumb:

Extension

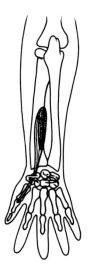

Position of m. extensor pollicis brevis

| | | $_{C6}$ | $_{C7}$ | $_{C8}$ | | | | M. extensor pollicis brevis

General comments

The basic movement is extension of the metacarpophalangeal joint of the thumb.

The starting position for all grades is maximal flexion with the forearm in pronation. The hand is held as an extension of the forearm.

The range of movement is limited by the structure of the joint and the ligaments of the palm.

Table 36.1

Prime mover	Origin	Insertion	Innervation
Extensor pollicis brevis	Third quarter of posterior surface of radius and adjacent interosseous membrane distal to abductor pollicis longus	Dorsal surface of base of proximal phalanx of thumb	Radial nerve (C6) C7 (C8)

Assisting muscles: Extensor pollicis longus

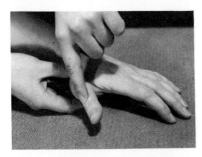

Grades 5, 4
Starting position: Supine lying or sitting with the forearm in pronation on the plinth and the hand as an extension of the forearm. The thumb is midway between adduction and abduction and flexed at the metacarpophalangeal joint, and the fingers are relaxed.
Fixation: The first metacarpal.
Movement: Extension of the metacarpophalangeal joint of the thumb.
Resistance: On the posterior aspect of the proximal phalanx of the thumb.

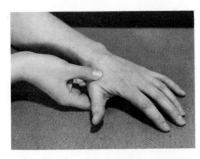

Grades 3–2
Starting position, fixation and movement: The same as for grades 5 and 4 without resistance.

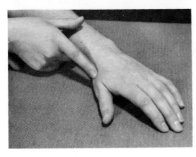

Grades 1, 0
Movement: The tendon of the extensor pollicis brevis is palpated at the base of the first metacarpal.

Possible errors

1. Movement does not occur at the metacarpophalangeal joint of the thumb.
2. During palpation there is confusion with the tendon of the extensor pollicis longus.

Shortening

Flexion of the metacarpophalangeal joint through the full range of movement is impossible when shortening is present.

37   The interphalangeal joint of the thumb:

Flexion

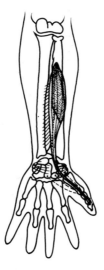

Position of m. flexor pollicis longus

| | | C6 | C7 | C8 | T1 | | | M. flexor pollicis longus

General comments

The basic movement is flexion of the interphalangeal joint of the thumb through a range of movement of 80 degrees.

The forearm is in supination during the test.

Fixation of the proximal phalanx is necessary to maintain the most favourable position.

Grades 3 and 2 are not differentiated.

The range of movement is limited by the structure of the joint.

Table 37.1

Prime mover	Origin	Insertion	Innervation
Flexor pollicis longus	Anterior aspect of radius between anterior oblique line and attachment of pronator quadratus and adjacent interosseous membrane	Palmar surface of base of distal phalanx of thumb	Median nerve (C6) C7 C8 (T1)

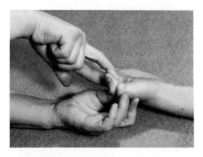

Grades 5, 4
Starting position: Supine lying or sitting. The forearm is in supination on the plinth. The thumb is extended and abducted and the fingers are relaxed.
Fixation: The proximal phalanx of the thumb, from both sides.
Movement: Flexion of the interphalangeal joint of the thumb through the full range of movement.
Resistance: Against the palmar aspect of the distal phalanx of the thumb.

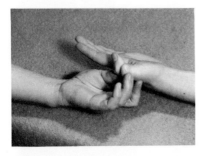

Grades 3–2
Starting position, fixation and movement: The same as grades 5 and 4, without resistance.

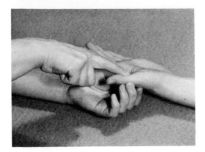

Grades 1, 0
Starting position: Supine lying or sitting with the forearm resting in supination on the plinth.
Fixation: The proximal phalanx of the thumb.
Movement: The movement of the tendon of the flexor pollicis longus can be palpated on the palmar aspect of the proximal phalanx of the thumb.

Possible errors

Errors are very rare.

Shortening

When this occurs the thumb is flexed at the interphalangeal joint.

38   The interphalangeal joint of the thumb:

Extension

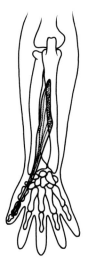

Position of m. extensor pollicis longus

| | | C6 | C7 | C8 | | | | M. extensor pollicis longus

General comments

The basic movement is extension from maximal flexion in the interphalangeal joint of the thumb.

In all grades the forearm is in pronation with the hand as an extension of the forearm. This extension of the wrist causes simultaneous relaxation of the extensor pollicis longus and makes the movement more difficult.

The range of movement is limited by the joint capsule.

Table 38.1

Prime mover	Origin	Insertion	Innervation
Extensor pollicis longus	Middle third of posterior surface of ulna and adjacent interosseous membrane distal to abductor pollicis longus	Dorsal aspect of base of distal phalanx of thumb	Radial nerve (C6) C7 (C8)

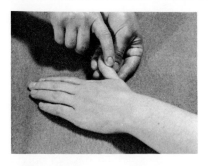

Grades 5, 4

Starting position: Supine lying or sitting with the forearm resting in pronation on the plinth. The thumb is flexed at the interphalangeal joint and extended at the metacarpophalangeal joint. The fingers are extended.
Fixation: The proximal phalanx from both sides.
Movement: Extension at the interphalangeal joint.
Resistance: Against the thumbnail.

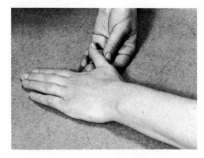

Grades 3—2

Starting position, fixation and movement: The same as grades 5 and 4, however without resistance

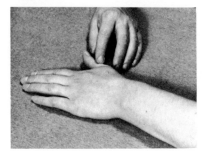

Grades 1, 0

Starting position: The forearm is in pronation on the plinth with the hand as an extension of the forearm.
Movement: The movement of the tendon of the extensor pollicis longus can be palpated on the posterior aspect of the distal phalanx of the thumb or the base of the first metacarpal posterolateral to the tendon of the extensor pollicis brevis.

Possible errors

1. Movement does not take place only at the interphalangeal joint and associated movements of the metacarpophalangeal joint or the wrist joint are allowed.
2. On palpation of the contraction there may be confusion with the tendon of the extensor pollicis brevis.

Shortening

This causes reduced flexion at the interphalangeal joint of the thumb.

Part 4   The lower limb

The lower limb has a similar structure to the upper one but is modified in accordance with its function of supporting and propelling the body. Thus its range of movement is not as large as that of the upper limb. The most important difference is in the connection of the femur with the pelvis, which has not only a large range of movement but also a weight-bearing capability. Another dissimilarity is the way the lower leg moves. The rotation that is so important in the forearm is almost non-existent in the lower leg. The third main difference is in the structure of the foot, which is primarily adapted to its supporting function and does not allow fine motor movements. Some of the muscles of the foot are very rudimentary and show regressive development.

The connection between the pelvis and the trunk is the hip joint. This is a ball-and-socket joint. The acetabulum covers two thirds of the femoral head and the range of movement is therefore relatively limited.

The main movements in the hip joint are as follows:

1. Flexion and extension, producing respectively forward and backward movement of the leg. Flexion has a range of movement of up to 120 degrees with the knee flexed. Hyperextension behind the frontal plane is only possible to 15 degrees.
2. Adduction and abduction which are the inward and outward movement of the leg respectively. The range of movement in each direction is 45 degrees.
3. Medial and lateral rotation. The range of medial rotation is 30 degrees and of lateral rotation is 45 degrees. This gives a full range of motion of 75 degrees. However, variations in the range of motion are great.

Through combinations of these main directions other movements, particularly circumduction, are possible.

The knee joint is made up of the femur and the tibia. On the front of the knee joint is a large sesamoid bone, namely the patella. The knee joint is the biggest joint in the body and possesses several joint surfaces and a number of ligaments. To improve the connection between the femur and the tibia the menisci are inside the joint; these decrease the unevenness between the surfaces. In the knee joint only one set of movements has practical importance, that is flexion and extension within the range 120–140 degrees. When the knee joint is flexed to 90 degrees and relaxed, rotation to 50–60 degrees can take place.

The ankle joint consists anatomically of two joints. First there is the upper ankle joint which is composed of the tibia, the fibula and the talus move. Secondly there is the lower ankle joint, consisting of the talus, the calcaneus and the navicular bones.

Besides these important joints the lower limb has a few others of less significance. The joints of the foot make one functional unit. Its main movements are the following:

1. Dorsiflexion and plantar flexion. The possible range of movement is 70 degrees, of which 40 degrees is plantar flexion and 30 degrees is dorsal flexion.
2. Eversion and inversion.
3. Supination and pronation.

The joints of the toes do not have such a large range of movement as do the joints of the fingers. Despite this, they are of great importance for keeping the balance when standing on tiptoe, walking, jumping and so on. In the metatarsophalangeal joints flexion and extension are possible and, to a lesser extent, adduction and abduction. Adduction and abduction are movements that are very seldom used by the human being. In the interphalangeal joints flexion and extension alone can take place.

The nerve supply of the lower limb

The innervation of the legs derives from two segments of two different plexuses, namely the lumbar and the sacral.

The lumbar plexus receives its main fibres from L1, L2 and L3 and also has connections to the nerve roots of T12 and L4. From it derive the muscular branches and the iliohypogastric, ilioinguinal, genitofemoral, lateral cutaneous, femoral and obturator nerves.

The lumbar branches innervate the quadratus lumborum, the psoas major and the psoas minor.

The iliohypogastric nerve (T12, L1) is a mixed nerve. It supplies the muscles of the trunk (the obliquus externus abdominis, the obliquus internus abdominis, the transversus abdominis and the rectus abdominis). Its main branches (the lateral cutaneous and anterior cutaneous nerves) innervate the pubic and hip areas.

The ilioinguinal nerve (T12–L1) innervates the transversus abdominis, and the obliquus internus abdominis provides a sensory supply to the inguinal area (in men to the scrotum and part of the penis and in women to the labia and part of the pubis).

The genitofemoral nerve (L1, L2) supplies the cremaster, the scrotum or the labia and a small area below the groin.

The lateral cutaneous nerve (L2, L3) is almost completely sensory. It innervates the skin on the lateral side of the thigh and the tensor fasciae latae.

Table P4.1 Femoralis nerve root innervation L1–L4. The position of nerve branches for particular muscles

Muscle	Site of branch
Iliopsoas	in the stomach close to the spina iliaca anterior superior
Sartorius	in the upper third of the upper thigh
Quadriceps (a) rectus	in the upper third of the upper thigh
(b) vastus lateralis (fibularis)	in the upper third of the upper thigh near the centre
(c) vastus medialis (tibialis)	in the upper third of the upper thigh
(d) vastus intermedius	in the upper third of the upper thigh
Pectineus	in the upper third of the upper thigh

    The femoral nerve (L1–L4) (*Table P4.1*) is the largest nerve in the lumbar plexus. This is a mixed nerve supplying the iliopsoas, the sartorius, the quadriceps femoris and the pectineus. The cutaneous fibres pass to the anteromedial side of the thigh and extend as the saphenous nerve to the anteromedial side of the

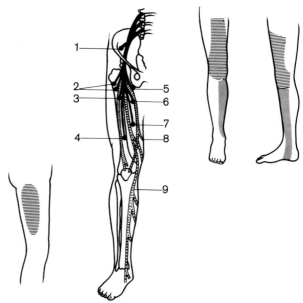

Sensitive area for n. cutaneus femoris lateralis
Schematic diagram of the course of n. femoralis (n. saphenus, n. cutaneus femoris anterior)
(1) m. iliacus, (2) m. rectus femoris, (3) m. vastus lateralis, (4) m. vastus intermedius, (5) m. pectineus, (6) m. sartorius, (7) m. vastus medialis, (8) n. cutaneus femoris anterior, (9) n. saphenus
Sensitive area for n. femoralis

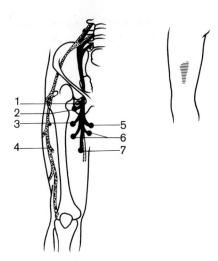

Schematic diagram of the course of n. obturatorius and n. cutaneus femoris lateralis
(1) m. pectineus, (2) m. obturatorius externus, (3) m. adductor magnus, (4) sensitive branch of n. obturatorius, (5) m. adductor longus, (6) m. adductor brevis, (7) m. gracilis
Sensitive area for n. obturatorius

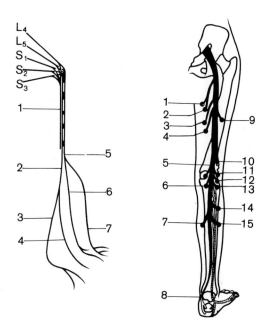

Schematic diagram of the course of n. ischiadicus
(1) to the hamstrings, (2) n. tibialis, (3) n. tibialis posterior, (4) n. suralis, (5) n. peroneus communis, (6) n. peroneus superficialis, (7) n. peroneus profundus
Course and innervation sites for n. ischiadicus (+ n. tibialis)
(1) m. adductor magnus, (2) m. semimembranosus, (3) m. semitendinosus, (4) m. biceps femoris (c. longum), (5) n. tibialis, (6) m. soleus, (7) m. flexor digitorum longus, (8) n. tibialis posterior, (9) m. biceps femoris (c. breve), (10) n. peroneus communis, (11) m. gastrocnemius, (12) m. plantaris, (13) m. popliteus, (14) m. tibialis posterior, (15) m. flexor hallucis longus

knee and the medial part of the calf and the foot. For a lesion of the femoral nerve there is always a great motor loss. Flexion in the hip joint and extension in the knee joint may be impossible depending on the level at which the lesion occurs. The sensitivity in the area still supplied is also affected.

The obturator nerve (L2–L4) innervates the pectineus, the adductor longus, the adductor brevis, the gracilis, the adductor magnus, the adductor minimus and the obturatorius externus. Its cutaneous fibres supply an area on the inside of the thigh.

The sacral plexus consists of the ischial pudendal and coccygeal plexuses.

The ischial plexus (*Table P4.2*, L4–S3) gives off direct muscular branches and the superior gluteal, inferior gluteal, posterior femoral cutaneous and sciatic nerves.

Regarding the muscular branches, the innervation of the quadratus femoris also supplies the gemellus inferior, the gemellus superior and the obturatorius internus.

The superior gluteal nerve (L4–S1) runs to the gluteus medius, the gluteus minimus and the tensor fasciae latae.

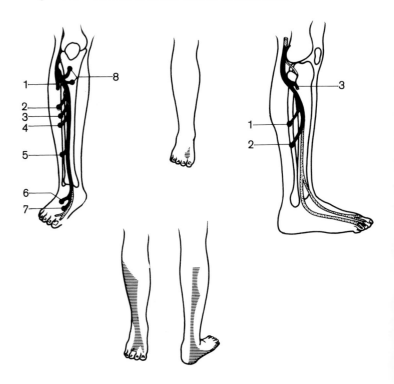

Innervation sites of n. peroneus profundus
(1) n. peroneus superficialis, (2) m. tibialis anterior, (3) m. extensor digitorum longus, (4) m. extensor hallucis longus, (5) m. peroneus tertius, (6) m. extensor digitorum brevis, (7) m. interosseus dorsalis I, (8) m. tibialis anterior
Sensitive area for n. peroneus profundus
Innervation sites for n. peroneus superficialis
(1) m. peroneus longus, (2) m. peroneus brevis, (3) n. peroneus profundus
Sensitive area for n. peroneus superficialis

Table P4.2   Plexus ischiadicus - root innervation L4–S3

Muscle	Branch
Adductor magnus	In the upper third of the upper thigh
Semimembranosus	In the upper third of the upper thigh
Semitendinosus	In the upper third of the upper half
Biceps femoris	In the upper half of the upper thigh

In the distal half of the upper thigh it divides into the N. tibialis and N. peroneus communis

N. tibialis
Triceps surae

(a) gastrocnemius	Upper half of the hollow of the knee
(b) soleus	In the hollow of the knee
Popliteus	In the hollow of the knee and at the head of the fibula
Plantaris	In the hollow of the knee
Tibialis posterior	In the upper third of the lower thigh
Flexor digitorum longus	In the upper third of the lower thigh
Flexor hallucis longus	In the upper third of the lower thigh

In the sole of the foot it divides into two branches, N. plantaris and N. plantaris lateralis

N. plantaris medialis

Abductor hallucis	On the sole of the foot
Flexor digitorum brevis	On the sole of the foot
Flexor hallucis brevis	On the sole of the foot
Lumbricales 1 and 2	On the sole of the foot

N. plantaris lateralis

Lumbricales 3 and 4	On the sole of the foot
Flexor hallucis brevis (caput laterale)	On the sole of the foot
Interossei plantares	On the sole of the foot
Adductor hallucis	On the sole of the foot

N. peroneus communis

Biceps femoris (caput breve)	In the middle of the upper thigh

At the head of the fibula this divides into

N. peroneus profundus

Tibialis anterior	In the proximal third of the lower thigh
Extensor digitorum longus	In the proximal half of the lower thigh
Extensor hallucis longus	In the middle of the lower thigh
Peroneus tertius	In the distal half of the lower thigh
Extensor digitorum brevis	On the back of the foot

N. peroneus superficialis

Peroneus longus	In the proximal half of the lower thigh
Peroneus brevis	In the middle of the lower thigh

The inferior gluteal nerve (L5–S2) innervates the gluteus maximus.

The posterior femoral cutaneous nerve (S1–S3) supplies the skin of the scrotum or labia, the buttocks and the upper and medial part of the thigh.

The sciatic nerve (L4–S3) is the largest nerve in the human body. In the thigh it supplies the biceps femoris, the semitendinosus, the semimembranosus and the ischial head of the adductor magnus. About halfway down the thigh it divides into two parts, namely the common peroneal and the tibial nerves.

The common peroneal nerve supplies the knee joint and as the lateral cutaneous nerve of the calf innervates the lateral surface of the calf. The sural nerve is composed of a branch from the tibial nerve. The common peroneal nerve later splits into the deep and superficial peroneal nerves. The former supplies the tibialis anterior, the extensor digitorum longus, the extensor digitorum brevis, the extensor hallucis longus and the extensor hallucis brevis. Its cutaneous branches innervate the lateral side of the big toe and the medial side of the second toe. The superficial peroneal nerve supplies the peroneus longus and the peroneus brevis and then divides into two parts which serve the skin of the top of the foot and the toes, except for one area innervated by the deep peroneal nerve.

In lesions of the common peroneal nerve the foot drops and dorsiflexion of the foot and the toes is impossible. The patient cannot stand on the heels and therefore the legs are bent more than normal in the hip and knee joints to avoid stumbling on the toes. In walking the sole of the foot slams noisily against the floor and the top of the foot, not the heel, touches the floor first. The whole foot is flat and passive movement increases considerably. The arch of the foot is diminished. This type of walking is often called a pigeon-gait. Sensitivity is decreased in the area supplied by the damaged nerve, that is on the lateral side of the calf and on top of the foot.

The tibial nerve gives off several branches. The most important before its final division are as follows:

1. Nerves to the gastrocnemius, the plantaris, the soleus, the popliteus, the tibialis posterior, the flexor digitorum longus and the flexor hallucis longus.
2. The sural nerve, which consists of branches of the tibial and deep peroneal nerves. This is a sensory nerve that innervates the posterior part of the lower leg, the lateral part of the heel and the lateral edge of the fifth toe.
3. Branches to the knee and the ankle joint.
4. Fibres to the skin on the medial side of the heel.

After this, the tibial nerve splits into two parts. The medial plantar nerve supplies the abductor hallucis, the flexor digitorum brevis, the flexor hallucis brevis and the first and second lumbricales pedis. Its cutaneous branch innervates the medial side of the foot and the plantar part of the first four toes. The lateral plantar nerve supplies the quadratus plantae, the flexor accessorius digitorum, the abductor digiti minimi pedis, the flexor digiti minimi brevis, the interossei dorsales pedis, the third and fourth lumbricales pedis and the adductor hallucis. Its cutaneous branch innervates the lateral side of the foot and the fourth and fifth toes.

In summary, the tibial nerve innervates the flexors, supinators, long flexors and in fact most of the muscles of the foot. It supplies the skin of the greater part of the heel and the sole.

In a lesion of the tibial nerve it may be impossible to stand on tiptoe and difficult to jump on one leg, depending on the level of the injury. Supination of the foot and flexion of the toes are impossible. Sensitivity is impaired in the heel and sole, excepting the lateral part.

The pudendal (S2–S4) and coccygeal plexuses (S5–C0) supply the skin of the genitals and the surrounding area.

The muscles of the lower limb

The muscles of the leg are similar to those of the arms, but have a different build and arrangement because of their double purpose of moving and weight bearing. While the muscles of the hands and fingers have special significance in the upper limb, the corresponding muscles of the foot are of secondary importance and some of them have been subject to regression.

There is a large muscle mass around the hip joint which gives both a wide range of movement and stability. Its influence on the position of the pelvis and the spine brings about the upright posture of the body.

There are two types of muscles in the hip joint, namely short muscles with a large cross section which are very strong, and long muscles that pass over the hip and knee joints and insert on the lower leg. The muscles of the hip joint tend to be divided into five functional groups, that is extensors on the posterior part, flexors on the anterior part, adductors on the inside of the thigh, abductors on the outside of the hip, and rotators that pass diagonally across the joint. The separate muscle groups do not have the same strengths and the weakest are situated where the ligaments of the joint are strongest and vice versa. The flexors are stronger than the extensors, the adductors are stronger than the abductors and the lateral rotators are three times as strong as the medial rotators.

On the posterior part of the hip joint the gluteal muscle group consists of the gluteus maximus, the gluteus medius, the gluteus minimus and the tensor fasciae latae. The gluteus maximus is considered the most important extensor of the hip joint, especially in extension posterior to the frontal plane. It assists adduction (the lower part), abduction (the upper part) and lateral rotation, and together with the tensor fasciae latae makes up the iliotibial tract. Its development is connected with the upright posture of the human being because it stabilizes the pelvis during walking when the leg is weight bearing in the standing phase, during walking up stairs and during standing up from sitting. The tensor fasciae latae participates in abduction, flexion and medial rotation of the hip joint. As part of the iliotibial tract it aids lateral rotation of the lower leg. The gluteus medius is mainly an abductor, but its anterior fibres contribute to flexion and medial rotation and its posterior fibres aid extension and lateral rotation of the hip joint. The gluteus minimus is synergistic with the gluteus medius and has practically the same function.

On the anterior part of the hip joint are the flexor muscles. These mainly comprise the iliopsoas, the sartorius, the rectus femoris and part of the tensor fasciae latae. The sartorius and the rectus femoris are two-joint muscles and contribute to both hip and knee joint movements. In addition the iliopsoas also acts during forward bending and lateral flexion of the spine.

The hip adductors consist of the adductor longus, the adductor brevis, the adductor magnus, the gracilis and the pectineus. The adductor magnus aids extension of the hip joint with its ischial head and lateral rotation with its pubic head. The medial part of the muscle, together with the gracilis, assists medial rotation. The pectineus, the adductor longus and the adductor brevis are not only adductors but also influence flexion and lateral rotation.

Six muscles laterally rotate the lower limb, that is the piriformis, the obturatorus externus, the obturatorus internus, the gemellus superior, the gemellus inferior and the quadratus femoris. Their function is lateral rotation, although other muscles of the hip joint may take part in the movement.

There is no special muscle group for medial rotation. The most important muscles for this movement are the gluteus minimus, the gluteus medius, the tensor fasciae latae and to a lesser extent the gracilis, the adductor magnus and the pectineus.

The abductors are a large muscle group comprising the tensor fasciae latae, the gluteus medius, the gluteus minimus and part of the gluteus maximus.

The muscles on the posterior part of the thigh are flexors of the knee joint, but with a fixed knee they also help extension of the hip joint. They consist of the biceps femoris, the semitendinosus and the semimembranosus. With the exception of the shortest head of the biceps femoris, they are all two-joint muscles originating from the ischial tuberosity and inserting on the lower leg. Therefore they are called ischiocrural muscles.

On the anterior side of the thigh, apart from those muscles already mentioned (the sartorius and the rectus femoris), there are three one-joint muscles of the knee joint, namely the vastus medialis, the vastus intermedius and the vastus lateralis. Together with the rectus femoris they form the quadriceps muscles. They all originate from one tendon which is inserted into the tibial tuberosity as the ligamentum patellae. The extensors are three times as strong as the flexors (the opposite situation holds true for the arm). This is to aid the upright posture of the body and assist the walking pattern.

The muscles of the lower leg fall into three groups, namely anterior, posterior and lateral.

Dorsiflexion of the foot is performed by the tibialis anterior, the extensor digitorum longus, the extensor hallucis longus and the peroneus tertius (in order of strength).

Plantar flexion is carried out by the gastrocnemius, the soleus, the flexor hallucis longus, the peroneus longus, the tibialis posterior, the flexor digitorum longus and the peroneus brevis. The plantar flexors are more than four times as strong as the dorsiflexors, which corresponds to their basic function of elevating the body during tiptoeing, walking, running and so on.

During inversion of the foot the muscles basically activated are the gastrocnemius, the soleus, the tibialis posterior, the flexor hallucis longus, the flexor digitorum longus and the tibialis anterior. For eversion the most active muscles are the peroneus longus, the peroneus brevis, the extensor digitorum longus, the peroneus tertius and the extensor hallucis longus. The inverters are twice as strong as the everters.

The short foot muscles are situated in the foot next to the tendons of the muscles of the lower leg. Compared with the muscles of the hand there are the following major differences:

1. There is no muscle corresponding to the opponens of the thumb.
2. The quadratus plantae does not have an equivalent in the hand.
3. The extensor digitorum brevis has no equivalent in the hand.
4. The lumbricales and interossei in the foot are rudimentary and subject to regression compared to those in the hand.

On the dorsum the short muscles of the foot are the extensor digitorum brevis and the extensor hallucis brevis. In the sole of the foot the short muscles are the flexor digitorum brevis, the quadratus plantae, the lumbricales pedis, the abductor hallucis, the flexor hallucis brevis, the adductor hallucis, the abductor digiti minimi pedis and the flexor digiti minimi brevis. These have not got the ability to perform fine movements like the short muscles of the hand. However, they are very important in walking because they help to provide the elasticity of the foot. Otherwise their significance is in their static function when keeping the balance. In this they are supported by a dense network of ligaments. The muscles and ligaments are much stronger on the inside than the outside of the foot.

To sum up, the lower limb possesses stability and at the same time a large range of movement.

39   The hip joint:

Flexion

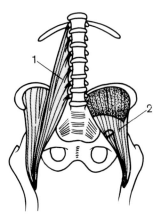

Position of the flexion muscles in the hip joint
(1) m. psoas major, (2) m. iliacus

| | | L1 | L2 | L3 | L4 | | M. psoas major |
| | | L1 | L2 | L3 | L4 | | M. iliacus |

General comments

The basic movement is flexion in the hip joint with a range of 120 degrees.

Grades 5, 4, 3, 1 and 0 are tested in a supine position and grade 2 in side lying. During the movement the pelvis must remain fixed and must not tilt backwards to produce lumbar kyphosis. In principle, supine lying is preferable as a starting position. When the trunk muscles are very strong the test can be done in the sitting position. However, this has the disadvantages that only the last 30 degrees of movement are tested and the examined muscle is in a position that does not allow the use of its full strength.

The pelvis must always be fixed even when it does not seem necessary; for example, when the trunk muscles are very strong.

If there is limited movement in the hip joint, extra care must be taken because patients often try to increase the range of movement by tilting the pelvis backwards. The movement should be performed smoothly at an even speed without any deviation in the sagittal plane.

The range of movement is limited by the joint structure.

Table 39.1

Prime mover	Origin	Insertion	Innervation
Iliopsoas psoas major	Superficial part: sides of vertebral bodies T12–L4	Lesser trochanter	Lumbar plexus femoral nerve (L1) L2 L3 (L4)
	Deep part: transverse processes L1–L5	Lesser trochanter	
iliacus	Iliac fossa	Lesser trochanter	(L1) L2 L3 (L4)

Assisting muscles: Pectineus, rectus femoris, tensor fasciae latae, gluteus minimus (anterior part), adductor brevis, sartorius, gluteus medius (anterior part), gracilis, adductor longus
Neutralizers: Tensor fasciae latae, pectineus
Stabilizers: Extensors of the lumbar spine and the abdominal muscles

Tests

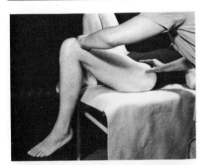

Grades 5, 4
Starting position: Supine lying with the lower leg over the end of the plinth and the foot unsupported. The other leg rests with a bent knee and a foot on the plinth. The arms rest by the sides.
Fixation: The pelvis is fixed over the anterosuperior iliac spine. The examiner stands by the side to be tested.
Movement: Flexion through the full range of movement.
Resistance: The examiner's hand is placed on the anterior aspect of the distal side of the thigh.

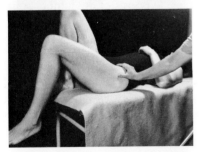

Grade 3
Starting position: Supine lying with the lower leg over the end of the plinth and the foot unsupported. The other leg has the hip and knee flexed and the foot supported on the plinth. The arms rest by the sides.
Fixation: The pelvis is fixed over the anterosuperior iliac spine.
Movement: Flexion in the hip joint.

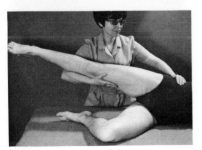

Grade 2
Starting position: Lying on the side of the tested leg with the hip in extension and the knee in flexion.
Fixation: The examiner fixes the pelvis with one hand and uses the other to support the untested leg in a slightly abducted position.
Movement: Flexion in the hip joint through the full range of movement.

161

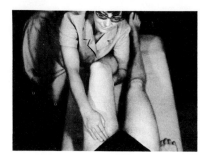

Grades 1, 0
Starting position: Supine lying.
Fixation: The examiner uses the forearm to support the lower part of the tested leg. The hip joint is semiflexed and laterally rotated to a slight extent with minimal knee flexion.
Movement: Contraction of the iliopsoas can be palpated just above the inguinal ligament medially to the sartorius.

Possible errors

1. Rotation of the whole leg is allowed and the movement does not only take place in the sagittal plane. Lateral rotation and abduction are a sign of either substitution of the sartorius or imbalance between the tensor fasciae latae, the sartorius and the adductors of the hip.
2. The movement is not done smoothly and the patient is allowed to jerk at its commencement.
3. The correct position of the pelvis is not observed and kyphosis of the lumbar spine is allowed. Fixation of the pelvis is therefore of great importance, especially when the trunk muscles are weak.
4. If the quadratus lumborum is too strong and overactive the patient tends to elevate the pelvis, especially at the beginning of the test.
5. If the patient compensates the movement by trunk flexion using the abdominal muscles, kyphosis of the lumbar spine occurs.

Shortening

This causes flexion of the hip joint and in standing there is exaggerated lordosis of the lumbar spine. The scoliosis is convex towards the side of the shortening to compensate for the apparent deficit in the leg.

40 The hip joint:

Extension

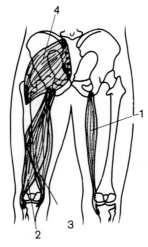

Position of the extensor muscles in the hip joint
(1) m. semitendinosus, (2) m. biceps femoris, (3) m. semimembranosus, (4) m. gluteus maximus

|	|	|L4	|L5	|S1	|S2	|	|	|	M. gluteus maximus
|	|	|	|L5	|S1	|S2	|S3	|	|	M. biceps femoris – caput longum
|	|	|L4	|L5	|S1	|S2	|	|	|	M. semitendinosus
|	|	|L4	|L5	|S1	|S2	|	|	|	M. semimembranosus

General comments

The basic movement is extension in the hip joint. With a bent knee the range of motion is 130–140 degrees. The full range is only tested in grade 2. Grades 5, 4 and 3 start the test with the hip joint in neutral so that the range of the movement is 10–15 degrees. However, this part of the range is very important in walking.

Extension of the hip joint presents a comparatively variable pattern, which is often altered with uneconomical results. In principle, if the patient is lying in supination three groups of muscles, namely the gluteus maximus, the hamstrings (which probably play a greater role than was earlier thought) and the paravertebral back muscles (which stabilize the lumbar spine and the pelvis) are activated. In many subjects the gluteus maximus is inhibited and the two other muscle groups take over

163

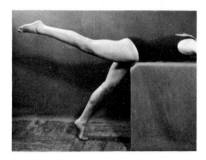

(a)

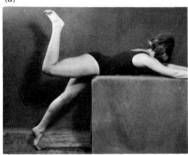

(b)

the performance of the movement. The torque is transferred to the lumbosacral angle and fixation of the pelvis is necessary. To gain a better evaluation the greater trochanter is palpated. If it slips during the test this proves that the movement is taking place in the hip joint.

The extension action of the gluteus maximus is decreased if the hip is in medial rotation and increased if it is in lateral rotation. To standardize the movement a constant position between lateral and medial rotation must be maintained. Estimation of the quality of the function of the gluteus maximus is necessary to explain many of the changes in motor disturbances. Because of this, the analysis must be exact. It is not possible to discern a tiny decrease of function by the classic tests, and therefore more detailed functional methods have been introduced to show better the variability or the weakness of the gluteus maximus.

In one modified test the patient is prone, lying with the trunk supported on the plinth and the hip joint flexed over the edge. The untested leg is steadied on the floor while the tested leg is lifted with the knee extended as high as possible (*Picture a*). With weakness of the muscle, the patient is not capable of lifting the leg above the horizontal and at the end of the movement abduction and/or medial rotation take place in the hip joint. The pattern is more clear when the test is performed with a flexed

Table 40.1

Prime mover	Origin	Insertion	Innervation
Gluteus maximus	Thoracolumbar fascia, sacrum, coccyx, sacrotuberous ligament, ilium (from iliac crest to posterior gluteal line)	Cranial part: gluteal tuberosity of femur Caudal part: iliotibial tract	Inferior gluteal nerve (L4) L5 S1 S2
Biceps femoris (long head)	Ischial tuberosity	Head of fibula, lateral condyle of tibia	Tibial part of sciatic nerve L5 S1 S2 (S3)
Semitendinosus	Ischial tuberosity	Converts with sartorius and gracilis into pes anserinus and inserts below medial condyle of tibia	Tibial part of sciatic nerve (L4) L5 S1 S2
Semimembranosus	Ischial tuberosity	Groove on medial condyle of tibia and posterior part of capsule of knee joint	Tibial part of sciatic nerve (L4) L5 S1 S2

Assisting muscles: Adductor magnus (fibres from ischial tuberosity), gluteus medius (posterior part), gluteus minimus (posterior part)
Neutralizers: Gluteus medius, adductors
Stabilizers: The abdominal muscles and the extensors of the lumbar spine

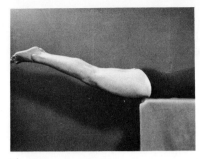

(c)

knee (*Picture b*). Usually in these tests no resistance is given because simple observation is more decisive.

In another test both legs are lifted at the same time without touching each other (*Picture c*). This makes it possible to judge the speed of lifting (the retardation phenomena), the symmetry of elevation and the final comparative positions of the legs. In an asymmetrical lesion the affected leg is lifted more slowly and not as high as the other. This test is very sensitive and should be introduced as a routine method.

The classic test of extension of the hip with a bent knee should not be excluded because in this case the hamstrings are under unfavourable conditions.

The range of movement is limited by the hip flexors (when the knee is flexed) and the iliofemoral ligament. When the hip flexors are shortened, they should all be tested before extension of the hip joint.

Tests

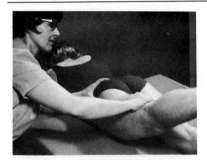

Grades 5, 4
Starting position: Prone lying with the legs in neutral and the feet over the edge of the plinth.
Fixation: The examiner's fingers and hand fix the pelvis of the tested side, while the thumb palpates the greater trochanter.
Movement: Extension at the hip joint 10–15 degrees behind the frontal plane.
Resistance: With the examiner's hand on the posterior aspect of the distal third of the thigh.

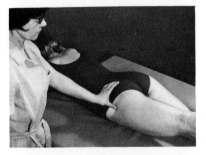

Grade 3
Starting position: Prone lying with the arms by the sides and the legs extended.
Fixation: The pelvis. The greater trochanter is palpated at the same time with the thumb.
Movement: Extension at the hip joint behind the frontal plane through a range of movement of 10–15 degrees.

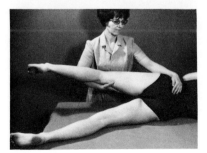

Grade 2
Starting position: Lying on the tested side. The untested leg is bent at the hip and knee joints and supported by the examiner. The tested leg is bent at the hip joint and extended at the knee joint.
Fixation: The pelvis at the superior iliac spine to avoid lordosis of the lumbar spine and to maintain slight abduction of the untested leg.
Movement: Extension at the hip joint through the full range of movement.

165

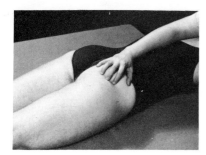

Grades 1, 0
Starting position: Prone lying with the legs extended.
Movement: Contraction of the gluteus maximus can be palpated within the muscle bulk. The other muscles can be palpated at their origins.

Selective test for gluteus maximus

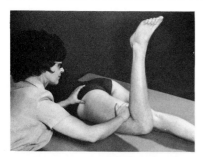

Grades 5,4
Starting position: Prone lying with the knee of the tested leg in flexion.
Fixation: The pelvis is fixed with the whole of the examiner's hand. The thumb palpates the greater trochanter.
Movement: Extension in the hip joint.
Resistance: Against the posterior aspect at the thigh.

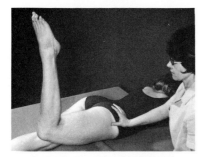

Grade 3
Starting position, fixation and movement: The same as for grades 5 and 4, but without resistance.

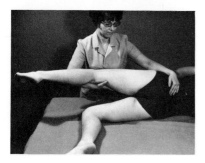

Grade 2
Starting position: Lying on the tested side. The untested leg is steadied by the examiner in flexion and slight abduction of the hip joint. The tested leg is flexed at the hip and knee joints.
Fixation: The superior iliac spine and the untested leg.
Movement: Extension through the full range of movement (130 degrees).

Possible errors

1. If fixation of the pelvis is overlooked a movement due to overactivity of the trunk erectors is allowed and the leg is lifted without extension at the hip joint. At the same time increased activity in the hamstrings becomes more evident.
2. If the correct position of the leg is overlooked rotation takes place.
3. The leg is adducted or abducted during the movement.

Shortening

In the gluteus maximus this is very rare. On the other hand, shortening of the hamstrings is common.

41 The hip joint:

Adduction

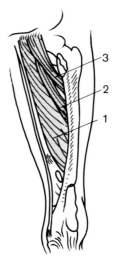

Position of the adductor muscles of the hip joint
(1) m. adductor magnus, (2) m. adductor longus, (3) m. adductor brevis

		L2	L3	L4	L5	S1			
		L2	L3	L4					M. adductor magnus
		L2	L3	L4					M. adductor longus
		L2	L3	L4					M. adductor brevis
		L2	L3	L4					M. gracilis
		L2	L3	L4					M. pectineus

General comments

The basic movement is adduction of the extended leg through a range of 30 degrees.

Grades 5, 4 and 3 are tested in lying on the side of the tested leg and grades 2, 1 and 0 in supine. It is important for the patient to lie correctly and to avoid backward or forward rotation. To keep this position the patient is allowed to stabilize the trunk with the hand on the plinth. When grades 2, 1 and 0 are tested the starting position is changed so that there is abduction to 30 degrees in the hip joint. It is incorrect to perform the movement with more abduction because this can cause displacement of the pelvis and facilitate or stretch the adductors too much.

The range of movement is limited by contact between the legs.

Table 41.1

Prime mover	Origin	Insertion	Innervation
Adductor magnus	In line with ischiopubic ramus and ischial tuberosity	Linea aspera (the medial supracondylar line to the medial epicondyle of the femur), tibial collateral ligament of the knee joint	Obturator nerve L3 L4 sciatic nerve L4 L5
Adductor longus	Small area of pubic bone below pubic tubercle	Middle part of medial lip of linea aspera	Obturator nerve L2 L3 (L4)
Adductor brevis	Below origin of adductor longus	Proximal third of medial lip of linea aspera	Obturator nerve L2 L3 L4
Gracilis	Lateral to pubic symphysis in line with inferior ramus of pubic bone	Pes anserinus on medial condyle of tibia	Obturator nerve L2 L3 L4
Pectineus	Pectineal line (pubic ligaments)	Line between lesser trochanter and linea aspera	Obturator nerve L2 L3 (L4) Femoral nerve L2 L3

Assisting muscles: Gluteus maximus (distal part), obturatorius externus and psoas major

Tests

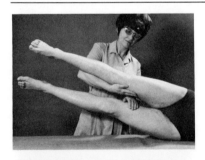

Grades 5, 4
Starting position: Side lying. The patient steadies the body on the edge of the plinth with the uppermost arm to fix the trunk. The other arm is placed under the head. The legs are extended and the tested leg is passively abducted to 30 degrees.
Fixation: To steady the untested leg in abduction.
Movement: Adduction of the leg towards the untested side.
Resistance: With the hand against the lower third of the thigh above the knee joint.

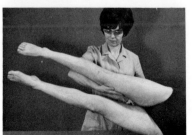

Grade 3
Starting position: Side lying. The patient steadies the trunk at the edge of the plinth with the uppermost arm while the other is placed under the head. The legs are extended and the untested leg is passively abducted to 30 degrees.
Fixation: The untested leg is held in 30-degrees abduction.
Movement: Adduction of the leg towards the untested side.

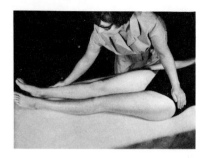

Grade 2
Starting position: Supine lying with both legs extended and abducted to 30 degrees.
Fixation: Not always necessary. The pelvis can be stabilized with one hand over the anterosuperior iliac spine.
Movement: Adduction of the leg about 10–15 degrees beyond the midline.

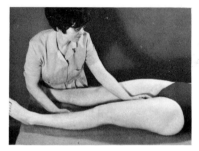

Grades 1, 0
Starting position: Supine lying, with the legs extended. The tested leg is slightly abducted.
Movement: Contraction of the adductors can be palpated on the inside of the thigh.

Possible errors

Faults are not common.

1.   If the trunk is in a position that allows rotation and flexion or slight hyperextension of the leg, other muscles can substitute for the movement.
2.   If the angle of abduction of the untested leg is not sustained, the position of the pelvis alters.

Shortening

The leg on the affected side looks shorter and, therefore, the opposite extremity in standing must be flexed or abducted or the patient has to stand on the toes of the affected side. In standing there is scoliosis convex towards the normal side. The range of hip abduction is limited.

42 The hip joint:

Abduction

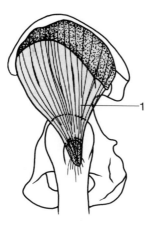

Position of m. gluteus medius

			L4	L5	S1	S2				M. gluteus medius
			L4	L5	S1	S2				M. tensor fasciae latae
			L4	L5	S1	S2				M. gluteus minimus

General comments

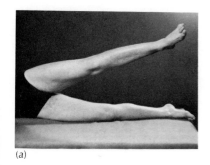

(a)

The basic movement is abduction through a range of 45 degrees.

Abduction together with extension is the most difficult movement of the hip joint and is altered very often in common postural defects, vertebragenic disease and so on. The gluteus medius and the gluteus minimus are the prime movers but the activity of the tensor fasciae latae and the iliopsoas should be remembered. If the last two muscles are dominant, the optimal pattern of abduction is compensated by lateral rotation and flexion in the hip joint. The pelvis is then rotated backwards and this allows even greater substitution (*Picture a*). This substitution can best be analysed by checking the level of the pelvis before the movement occurs.

During the test it is important for the patient to be in a position of side lying rather than slight forward rotation. A tendency to backward rotation of the trunk is a disadvantage. True abduction of the hip joint takes place without any movement of the pelvis. Elevation of the pelvis stresses the activity of the quadratus lumborum so that movement occurs in the lumbosacral region.

Fixation of the pelvis before the test starts is thus very important. At the same time the greater trochanter is palpated with the thumb and if it is felt to slip away this proves movement is taking place in the hip joint.

The range of movement is limited by the iliofemoral ligament, the pubofemoral ligament and the adductors of the hip joint.

Table 42.1

Prime mover	Origin	Insertion	Innervation
Gluteus medius	Outer surface of ilium between middle and posterior gluteal lines	Greater trochanter	Superior gluteal nerve L4 L5 S1 (S2)
Tensor fasciae latae	Outer surface of anterosuperior iliac spine	Iliotibial tract (inserts on lateral condyle of tibia)	Superior gluteal nerve L4 L5 S1 (S2)
Gluteus minimus	Outer surface of ilium between superior and inferior gluteal lines	Greater trochanter (anterior surface)	Superior gluteal nerve L4 L5 S1 (S2)

Assisting muscles: Piriformis
Neutralizers: The glutei equalize the reciprocal rotation components
Stabilizers: Quadratus lumborum (especially against resistance), back extensors and abdominal muscles

Tests

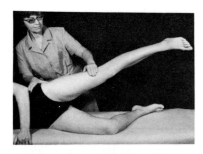

Grades 5, 4
Starting position: Lying on the untested side. The untested leg is slightly flexed at the hip and knee joints. The tested leg is extended at the knee joint and slightly hyperextended at the hip joint. The bottom arm should be in a comfortable position under the head. The other is in front of the body and the patient holds on to the edge of the plinth with it to stabilize the trunk.
Fixation: The examiner's whole hand on the tested side of the anterosuperior iliac spine. At the same time palpation of the greater trochanter checks that the correct movement is taking place.
Movement: Abduction of the extended leg through the full range of movement.
Resistance: From the examiner's hand on the outside of the lower third of the thigh.

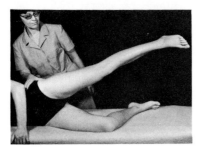

Grade 3
Starting position: Side lying. The untested leg is in half flexion. The tested leg at extended at the knee joint and slightly hyperextended at the hip joint. The bottom arm is underneath the head and the other stabilizes the trunk by grasping the edge of the plinth.
Fixation: The examiner's whole hand on the anterosuperior iliac spine of the tested side. At the same time palpation of the greater trochanter checks that the correct movement is taking place.
Movement: Abduction of the leg through the full range of movement.

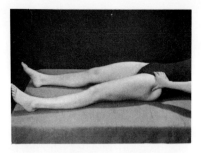

Grade 2
Starting position: Supine lying with the legs extended.
Fixation: On the tested side, the examiner keeps the fingers on the anterosuperior iliac spine. At the same time the thumb palpates the greater trochanter in order to check that the movement is being performed correctly.
Movement: Abduction in the hip joint through the full range of movement.

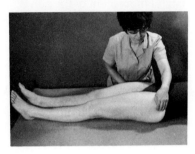

Grades 1, 0
Starting position: Supine lying with the legs extended.
Movement: The muscle contraction can be palpated at the greater trochanter.

Possible errors

1. If the pelvis is not fixed, substitution is possible through elevation of the pelvis. This can be detected in grades 5, 4 and 3 when a line between the anterosuperior iliac spines is not vertical to the horizontal.
2. Lateral rotation and flexion are allowed in the hip joint if the iliopsoas and the tensor fasciae latae take the role of prime movers.
3. Palpation of the greater trochanter is omitted.
4. Movement does not occur through the full range and resistance is not given in the right direction.

Shortening

This is noticeable in standing because the affected side of the pelvis is lowered and there is apparent lengthening of the leg. The latter is compensated through scoliosis of the lumbar spine convex towards the side of the contracture.

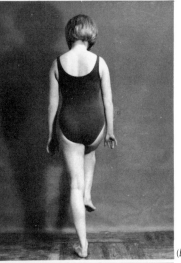

Note

In practice the examiner must be able to detect very slight deviations that can hardly be perceived by classic muscle tests. In these cases a refinement of the Trendelenburg test is recommended. This is positive not only when there is lowering of the pelvis but also when there is a lateral pelvic shift without lowering. The pelvis must be fixed before the patient stands on one leg and an attempt must be made to avoid laterally shifting it at the beginning of the test. Standing on one leg should be carried out without almost any lateral movement of the pelvis, at least within the first 20 seconds (*Picture b*). The examiner must check that the patient does not lift the pelvis at the same time as taking the leg off the floor (*Picture c*) or wrongly keep the balance by side-bending the trunk (*Picture d*). The lifted leg must be flexed to 90 degrees in the hip and knee joints. This test is very sensitive but assumes strong coordinated leg and trunk muscles.

(b)

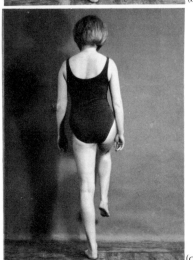

(c)

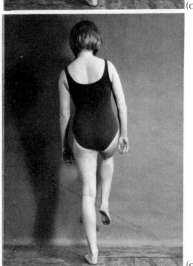

(d)

174

43 The hip joint:

Lateral rotation

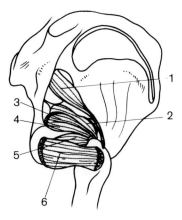

Position of the lateral rotation muscles in the hip joint
(1) m. piriformis, (2) m. gemellus superior, (3) m. obturatorius internus, (4) m. gemellus inferior, (5) m. obturatorius externus, (6) m. quadratus femoris

L3	L4	L5	S1	S2	S3	Muscle
	L4	L5	S1			M. quadratus femoris
		L5	S1	S2	S3	M. piriformis
	L4	L5	S1	S2		M. gluteus maximus
	L4	L5	S1	S2	S3	M. gemellus superior (spinalis)
	L4	L5	S1	S2		M. gemellus inferior (tuberalis)
L3	L4	L5				M. obturatorius externus
		L5	S1	S2	S3	M. obturatorius internus

General comments

The basic movement is lateral rotation through a range of 45 degrees.

All grades are noted supine. With grades 5, 4 and 3 the tested leg hangs free over the edge of the plinth. The other leg is bent with the foot steadied on the plinth to stabilize the pelvis. Grades 2, 1 and 0 are tested with outstretched legs. Grade 2 can be tested from two starting positions, namely supine and standing. The latter is less suitable because the patient has to activate the muscles of the trunk, mainly the quadratus lumborum, and also the whole tested leg.

Fixation of the lower third of the spine is necessary in grades 5, 4 and 3. When the patient tries to compensate for weakened muscles by lifting the pelvis, this must be fixed at the anterosuperior iliac spine.

The range of movement is limited by the iliofemoral ligament and the medial rotators of the hip joint.

Table 43.1

Prime mover	Origin	Insertion	Innervation
Quadratus femoris	Ischial tuberosity (outer border)	Intertrochanteric crest	Sacral plexus (L4) L5 S1
Piriformis	Anterior surface of sacrum along borders of second to fourth sacral foramina	Upper border of greater trochanter	Sacral plexus (L5) S1 S2 (S3)
Gluteus maximus	Thoracolumbar fascia, sacrum, coccyx, sacrotuberous ligament, gluteal surface of ilium, iliac crest, posterior gluteal line	Cranial part: gluteal tuberosity of femur Caudal part: iliotibial tract	Inferior gluteal nerve (L4) L5 S1 S2
Gemellus superior	Ischial spine	Trochanteric fossa	Sacral plexus (L4) L5 S1 S2 (S3)
Gemellus inferior	Ischial tuberosity	Trochanteric fossa	Sacral plexus (L4) L5 S1 (S2)
Obturatorius externus	Outer surface of obturator membrane, obturator foramen	Trochanteric fossa	Obturator nerve L3 L4 (L5)
Obturatorius internus	Pelvic surface of obturator membrane, obturator foramen	Trochanteric fossa	Sacral plexus (L5) S1 S2 (S3)

Assisting muscles: Adductor brevis, adductor longus, adductor magnus, gluteus medius (posterior part), pectineus, biceps femoris
Neutralizers: The individual muscles neutralize themselves
Stabilizers: Quadratus lumborum, abdominal muscles and back extensors

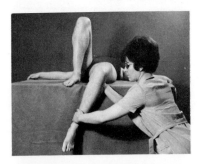

Grades 5, 4
Starting position: Supine lying. The tested leg hangs over the edge of the plinth. The other leg is bent with the foot steadied on the plinth.
Fixation: The lower third of the thigh at the back of the knee.
Movement: Medial rotation of the thigh through the full range of movement (45 degrees). The foot moves inwards.
Resistance: With the examiner's hand just above the medial malleolus.

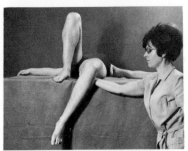

Grade 3
Starting position: Supine lying. The tested leg hangs over the edge of the plinth. The other leg is bent and steadied with the foot on the plinth.
Fixation: The lower third of the thigh at the back of the knee.
Movement: Lateral rotation at the hip joint through the full range of movement.

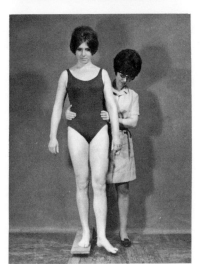

Grade 2a
Starting position: Standing on the untested leg on the floor or preferably on a low stool. The tested leg is slightly medially rotated and not touching the floor.
Fixation: The pelvis at the anterosuperior iliac spine.
Movement: Lateral rotation at the hip joint through the full range of movement.

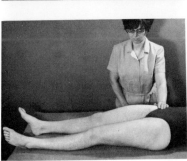

Grade 2b
Starting position: Supine lying with the legs extended. The tested leg is medially rotated.
Fixation: The pelvis is steadied on the untested side at the anterosuperior iliac spine.
Movement: Lateral rotation at the hip joint through the full range of movement. The crucial part of the test is the first section, that is from medial rotation to the midposition.

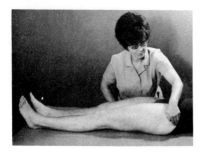

Grades 1, 0
Starting position: Supine lying with the legs extended.
Movement: Muscle contraction is palpated above the greater trochanter. The examiner must observe whether the leg attempts to move into lateral rotation.

Possible errors

1. In standing during the test for grade 2 the pelvis is not stabilized properly and there is elevation of the pelvis by the quadratus lumborum.
2. When testing grade 2 in supine lying, the patient imitates rotation by pronating the foot.

Shortening

This causes lateral rotation of the thigh which increases especially with abduction. The muscle most often shortened is probably the piriformis.

44 The hip joint:

Medial rotation

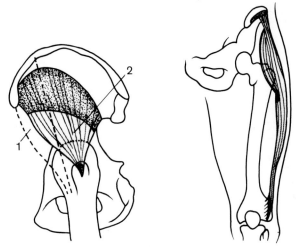

Position of the medial rotation muscles in the hip joint
(1) m. tensor fasciae latae, (2) m. gluteus minimus
Position of m. tensor fasciae latae

			L4	L5	S1	S2				M. gluteus minimus
			L4	L5	S1	S2				M. tensor fasciae latae

General comments

The basic movement is medial rotation through a range of 30 degrees.

All grades are tested supine. In grades 5, 4 and 3 the tested leg hangs free over the edge of the plinth while in the other grades the legs are extended. The untested leg is bent and the foot is steadied on the plinth. Thus hyperextension of the lumbar spine and tilting of the pelvis are eliminated. Grade 2 can also be tested in standing. However, in this position other muscles, including the quadratus lumborum, the abdominal muscles and the other leg muscles, are excessively activated.

With grades 5, 4 and 3 fixation above the knee joints is necessary. With grades 2, 1 and 0 the pelvis is usually fixed to avoid uncoordinated movements and elevation of the pelvis on the ipsilateral side.

The range of movement is limited by the lateral rotators of the hip joint, by the lower part of the iliofemoral ligament with the hip joint in extension and by the ischiofemoral ligament with the hip joint in flexion.

Table 44.1

Prime mover	Origin	Insertion	Innervation
Gluteus minimus	Outer surface of ilium between superior and inferior gluteal lines	Greater trochanter (anterior surface)	Superior gluteal nerve L4 L5 S1 (S2)
Tensor fasciae latae	Outer surface of anterosuperior iliac spine	Iliotibial tract (on lateral condyle of tibia)	Superior gluteal nerve L4 L5 S1 (S2)

Assisting muscles: Gluteus medius (anterior part), semitendinosus, gracilis, semimembranosus
Neutralizers: Adductor magnus counteracts the abduction component
Stabilizers: Quadratus lumborum, back extensors, abdominal muscles

Tests

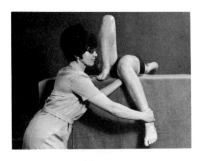

Grades 5, 4
Starting position: Supine lying. The tested leg is bent at the knee joint and the lower part hangs free over the plinth edge. The untested leg is bent at the knee joint with the foot steadied on the plinth.
Fixation: The lower third of the thigh.
Movement: Medial rotation at the hip joint through the full range of movement (30 degrees). The foot moves outwards.
Resistance: Above the lateral malleolus.

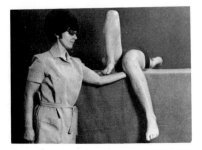

Grade 3
Starting position: Supine lying. The tested leg hangs free over the edge of the plinth. The untested leg is bent with the foot steadied on the plinth.
Fixation: The lower side of the thigh.
Movement: Medial rotation in the hip joint through the full range of movement.

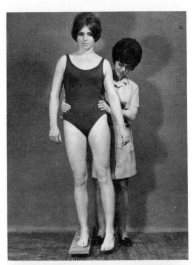

Grade 2a
Starting position: Standing on the untested leg, either on the floor or on a low stool. The tested leg is slightly laterally rotated and not touching the floor.
Fixation: Both the examiner's hands are placed on the anterosuperior iliac spines to stabilize the pelvis.

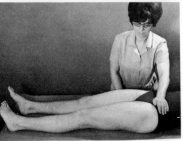

Grade 2b
Starting position: Supine lying. Both legs are extended. The tested leg is laterally rotated.
Fixation: With the examiner's hand lightly on the anterosuperior iliac spine of the tested side.
Movement: Medial rotation at the hip joint through the full range of movement.

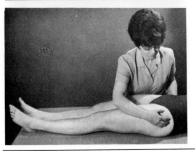

Grades 1, 0
Starting position: Supine lying.
Movement: Muscle contraction can be palpated above the greater trochanter.

Possible errors

1. The pelvis is not fixed and the correct position of the thigh is not retained in grades 5, 4 and 3.
2. In grades 2, 1 and 0 the patient tries to imitate the movement by adduction at the hip joint, sometimes combined with supination of the foot.
3. When the tensor fasciae latae is dominant the patient starts the medial rotation by slight flexion in the hip joint.

Shortening

This produces medial rotation of the thigh and a tendency to genu valgum. If, in addition, there is shortening of the tensor fasciae latae a flexion-abduction position of the hip joint also occurs.

45 The knee joint:

Flexion

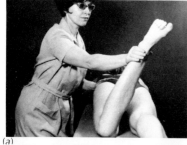

(a)

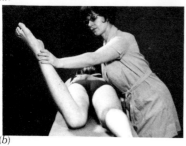

(b)

		L5	S1	S2	S3		M. biceps femoris – caput longum
	L4	L5	S1	S2			M. biceps femoris – caput breve
	L4	L5	S1	S1			M. semitendinosus
	L4	L5	S1	S2			M. semimembranosus

General comments

The basic movement is flexion at the knee joint through a range of 120–140 degrees. Grades 5, 4, 3, 1 and 0 are tested in prone lying.

During routine assessment the leg is kept in a position between medial and lateral rotation. It is advisable to use starting positions that make it possible to differentiate the medial and lateral hamstrings. If the hip joint is laterally rotated (*Picture a*), the lateral hamstrings (the biceps femoris) are more active. If the hip joint is medially rotated (*Picture b*), the medial hamstrings

Table 45.1

Prime mover	Origin	Insertion	Innervation
Biceps femoris	Long head: ischial tuberosity Short head: lateral lip of linea aspera (distal part)	Head of fibula, lateral condyle of tibia	Tibial part of sciatic nerve L5 S1 S2 (S3) Peroneal part of sciatic nerve (L4) L5 S1 S2
Semitendinosus	Ischial tuberosity	Converts with sartorius and gracilis into pes anserinus and inserts below medial condyle of tibia	Tibial part of sciatic nerve (L4) L5 S1 S2
Semimembranosus	Ischial tuberosity	Groove on medial condyle of tibia and posterior part of knee joint capsule	Tibial part of sciatic nerve (L4) L5 S1 S2

Assisting muscles: Gracilis, sartorius, popliteus, gastrocnemius
Neutralizers: Biceps femoris on one side and flexors on the opposite side
Stabilizers: Flexors of the hip joint

(the semimembranosus and the semitendinosus) work as prime movers. During the test the pelvis must not tilt forwards.

The range of movement may be limited by the ligamentum patellae (the tendon of the quadriceps femoris), that is the tightening of the rectus femoris, and the anterior part of the joint capsule. Normally motion is only limited by soft-tissue contact.

Tests

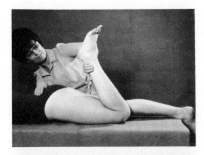

Grades 5, 4
Starting position: Prone lying. The legs are extended and the feet hang over the edge of the plinth.
Fixation: The pelvis is fixed by the whole of the examiner's hand.
Movement: Flexion at the knee joint through the full range of movement.
Resistance: With the examiner's hand on the distal third of the lower leg above the Achilles tendon.

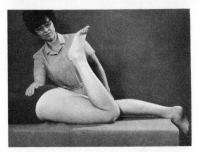

Grade 3
Starting position: Prone lying with the legs extended and the feet over the edge of the plinth.
Fixation: The pelvis by the whole of the examiner's hand.
Movement: Flexion through the full range of movement.

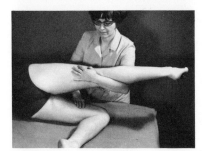

Grade 2
Starting position: Lying on the tested side. The untested leg is steadied in extension and slightly abducted at the hip joint.
Fixation: Slight resistance of the hand against the lower third of the inside of the thigh.
Movement: Flexion in the knee joint through the full range of movement.

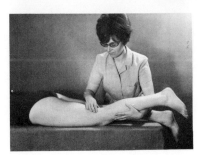

Grades 1, 0
Starting position: Prone lying. The untested leg is extended and the tested leg is slightly flexed at the knee joint and steadied at lower third of the lower leg.
Movement: Muscle contraction can be palpated within the muscle fibres or along the tendons.

Possible errors

1. In doubtful cases it is often necessary to differentiate between the lateral and medial knee flexors (see above).
2. At the beginning of the movement, if the patient lifts the pelvis the starting position changes to slight flexion in the hip and knee joints. This stretches the hamstrings and increases their activity. This can be eliminated by fixation of the pelvis.
3. Substitution by the sartorius causes flexion and lateral rotation of the hip joint. This starting position makes the test easier because it is not performed at right angles to the weight of the leg.

Shortening

This is common. In more severe cases extension of the knee joint is not possible, the pelvis is tilted backwards in the sagittal plane and there is flattening of the lumbar curve. With the most severe shortening the knee joint retains a flexion deformity. Predominant shortening of the biceps tendons can lead to genu valgum. If slight shortening is present, flexion of the hip joint to more than 80 degrees by simultaneously extending the knee is not possible (Pseudolassegue sign).

46   The knee joint:

Extension

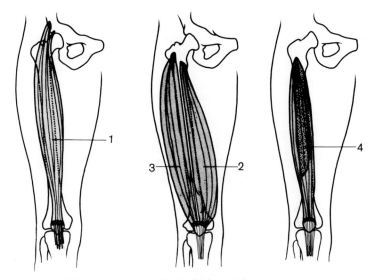

Position of the extension muscles in the knee joint
(1) m. rectus femoris, (2) m. vastus medialis, (3) m. vastus lateralis, (4) m. vastus intermedius

| | L2 | L3 | L4 | L5 | | | M. quadriceps femoris |

General comments

The basic movement is extension in the knee joint through a range of movement of 120–140 degrees. Only movement through the the last 90 degrees is assessed.

Grades 5, 4 and 3 are evaluated supine while the tested leg hangs freely over the edge of the plinth. The sitting position is less suitable, because with hip flexion the rectus femoris cannot work to its full strength. The untested leg is flexed with the foot steadied on the plinth so that the pelvis is stabilized. Grade 2 is tested in side lying and grades 1 and 0 in supine lying.

Fixation of the knee is always necessary, especially in children, to prevent rotation of the thigh and substitution by other muscles. Additionally, fixation of the leg is very important. The thigh must be steadied from underneath so as not to press on the quadriceps femoris.

The range of movement is limited by the cruciate and collateral ligaments and by the posterior part of the capsule.

Table 46.1

Prime mover	Origin	Insertion	Innervation
Quadriceps femoris:	Anteroinferior iliac spine above acetabulum	Base of patella and its borders, finally as ligamentum patellae on tibial tubercle	Femoral nerve (L2) L3 L4 (L5)
Rectus femoris	Groove above brim of acetabulum		
Vastus intermedius	Along the whole femur except linea aspera		
Vastus medialis (tibialis)	Medial lip of linea aspera		
Vastus lateralis (fibularis)	Lateral lip of linea aspera		

Stabilizers and neutralizers: Vastus lateralis and vastus medialis compensate lateral and medial components, hip extensors counteract flexion components of rectus femoris

Tests

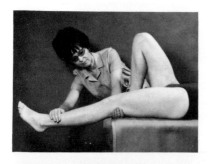

Grades 5, 4
Starting position: Supine lying. The lower part of the tested leg hangs freely over the edge of the plinth with the knee joint flexed to 90 degrees. The other leg is flexed with the foot steadied on the plinth.
Fixation: Posterior part of the thigh.
Movement: Extension in the knee joint from 90 degrees of flexion to full extension.
Resistance: Just above the malleoli.

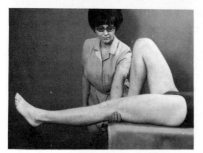

Grade 3
Starting position: Supine lying. The lower part of the tested leg lies over the edge of the plinth with the knee joint flexed to 90 degrees.
Fixation: Posterior part of the thigh.
Movement: From 90 degrees of flexion to full extension.

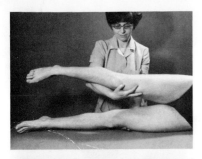

Grade 2

Starting position: Lying on the tested side. The other leg is extended at the knee joint and abducted slightly at the hip joint with the thigh and lower leg steadied. The tested leg is flexed at 90 degrees at the knee and the hip joint is kept in the line of trunk (zero position).

Fixation: The examiner's hand on the outside of the thigh just above the knee.

Movement: From 90 degrees of flexion to full extension.

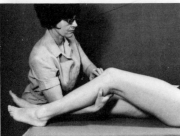

Grades 1, 0

Starting position: Supine lying with the untested leg extended. The tested leg is in semiflexion in the knee and hip joints and the knee is steadied lightly with one hand.

Movement: Palpation is carried out by the examiner's free hand over the ligamentum patellae and along the quadriceps femoris.

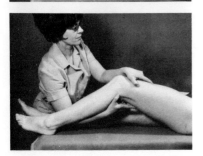

Possible errors

This movement is very simple and errors seldom occur.

1. The movement is carried out unevenly with the patient rushing the start.
2. There is rotation in the hip joint.
3. The pelvis tilts backwards if the test is taking place in sitting. A backward tilt is a sign that the rectus femoris is not strong enough or the hamstrings are shortened.
4. The movement is not carried out to full extension. If the patient cannot extend the knee fully, this is an indication of decreased strength of the vasti.
5. The thigh is fixed ventrally causing pressure on the quadriceps femoris.

Shortening

This is very common, especially shortening of the rectus femoris. It is manifested by decreased flexion at the knee joint, which is more marked prone with the hip joint fully extended. Complete extension of the hip joint is not possible when the knee is flexed.

187

47   The ankle joint:

Plantar flexion

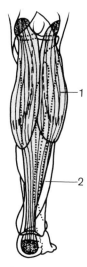

The muscles involved in plantar flexion of the ankle joint
(1) m. gastrocnemius, (2) m. soleus

					S1	S2			M. gastrocnemius
				L5	S1	S2			M. soleus

General comments

The basic movement is plantar flexion at the ankle joint with the knee extended. The range of movement is 40–45 degrees.

Grades 5, 4 and 3 are tested in prone lying and are distinguished by different resistances. Exact discrimination is very difficult. Grades 2, 1 and 0 are assessed in lying on the tested side. Grades 5, 4 and 3 can also be tested in standing, when the patient goes up on tiptoe. For grade 5 it must be possible to repeat this four or five times and for grade 4 at least once. In grade 3 the heel must lift from the floor. Because this assessment requires a lot of muscles to be activated it has many drawbacks and is not recommended. When the movement is performed in prone lying there are also drawbacks, especially if the resistance given by the examiner's hand is too slight in grade 5.

In plantar flexion the peroneus brevis, the peroneus longus, the tibialis posterior and the plantaris are activated. Their

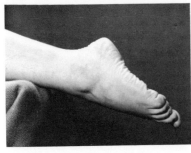

(a)

contribution cannot be eliminated while the movement is taking place, but through meticulous observation predominance of one or other muscle group can be estimated. The activity of the gastrocnemius is decreased when plantar flexion is tested with the knee flexed. This starting position is used to test the soleus as described below.

The motion due to the soleus and the gastrocnemius mainly takes place in the talocrural joint. It must be performed by moving the heel upwards and not by downward movement of the forefoot. If the forefoot and the toes are flexed, or even if the sole of the foot is "rolling up", this is a sign that the assisting muscles are working (*Picture a*). If the toes are flexed too much the toe flexors are being used. When there is supination at the same time, this is due to dominance of the anteriorly situated muscles while pronation is due to activity of the peroneal muscles.

The gastrocnemius and the soleus are tested together with the knee extended. The range of movement is limited partly by the ligament on the anterior part of the ankle joint but mainly by contact between the talus and the tibia dorsally.

Table 47.1

Prime mover	Origin	Insertion	Innervation
Gastrocnemius	Medial head (tibial): medial condyle of femur (dorsal part) Lateral head (fibular): lateral condyle of femur	Unites with soleus to form Achilles tendon (tendo calcaneus) which inserts into tubercle of calcaneum	Branch of tibial nerve S1 S2
Soleus	Head of fibula (posterior surface): proximal third of posterior surface of fibula, popliteal line and middle third of medial border of tibia	Unites with gastrocnemius to form Achilles tendon (tendo calcaneus) which inserts into tubercle of calcaneum	Branch of tibial nerve (L5) S1 S2

Assisting muscles: Tibialis posterior, plantaris, peroneus brevis, flexor hallucis longus, peroneus longus, flexor digitorum longus
Neutralizers: The peronei and the tibialis posterior both counteract the tendency to inversion and eversion of the foot
Stabilizers: None in lying

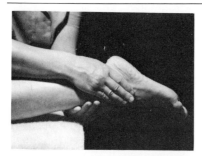

Grades 5, 4 3
Starting position: Prone lying. The legs are extended with the distal half of the lower leg over the edge of the plinth. The foot is fully relaxed.
Fixation: The distal third of the lower leg.
Movement: Plantar flexion at the ankle joint through the full range of movement.
Resistance: The heel is grasped by the examiner's hand and at the same time moved in a distal direction. The grades are separated by different resistances. The toes must not be flexed.

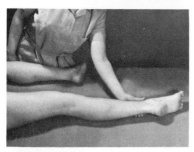

Grade 2
Starting position: Side lying on the side of the tested leg with the hip and knee joints in extension. The foot is flexed to 90 degrees and rests on its outside edge. The untested leg is in flexion.
Fixation: The distal third of the lower leg.
Movement: Plantar flexion through the full range of movement. The lateral side of the foot slides along the plinth.

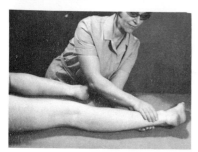

Grades 1, 0
Starting position: Lying on the tested side.
Movement: The Achilles tendon and gastrocnemius fibres can be palpated.

Possible errors

1. Movement does not take place very precisely, the heel does not move in a cranial direction and the forefoot is plantar flexed.
2. If the test takes place in standing, flexion in the knee joint occurs. It is possible to lift the heel from the floor even without movement in the talocrural joint with a slight forwards movement of the knee.

Shortening

With shortening, even passive dorsiflexion in the ankle joint from 90 degrees is not possible. In severe cases the patient cannot take the full weight on the whole foot and the foot is in the equinus position whether weight bearing or not.

48 The ankle joint:

Plantar flexion (soleus)

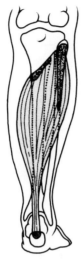

Position of m. soleus

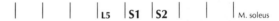

| | | | L5 | S1 | S2 | | | | M. soleus

General comments

The basic movement is plantar flexion of the foot with the knee in flexion. The range of motion is 40–45 degrees.

During examination of the soleus the same principles apply as to the combined test of the gastrocnemius and soleus. All the remarks regarding tests of the whole triceps surae are valid for isolated testing of the soleus.

Grades 5, 4 and 3 are tested either prone with the knee in flexion or in sitting. Grades 2, 1 and 0 are assessed while the patient is lying on the side of the tested leg. The standing position is not suitable. In sitting, the patient must be able to perform the movement against maximal resistance at least three times for grade 5 and once for grade 4, and against light resistance once for grade 3.

Substitution is common. The patient tries to extend the knee to activate the gastrocnemius. This is one reason why the standing position is not recommended. Testing of the soleus in standing with the knee flexed is unreliable because of the contraction of the leg muscles, and there is also a high risk of the patient losing balance and falling down.

The range of movement is limited by contact between the talus and the tibia, the ligaments on the anterior part of the ankle joint and stretching of the foot extensors.

Table 48.1

Prime mover	Origin	Insertion	Innervation
Soleus	Head of fibula (posterior surface), proximal third of posterior surface of fibula, popliteal line, middle third of medial border of tibia	Tubercle of calcaneum	Tibial nerve L5 S1 S2

Assisting muscles: Gastrocnemius, tibialis posterior, peroneus longus, peroneus brevis, flexor digitorum longus, flexor hallucis longus
Neutralizers: The peronei and the tibialis posterior counteract the tendency to inversion and eversion of the foot
Stabilizers: None in lying

Tests

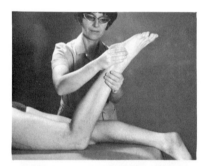

Grades 5a, 4a, 3a
Starting position: Prone lying with tested leg flexed at the knee joint.
Fixation: The distal half of the lower leg.
Movement: Plantar flexion through the full range of movement. The toes must not be flexed at the same time.
Resistance: The Achilles tendon is grasped by the examiner's fingers and the heel moved distally. The grades are separated by different resistances.

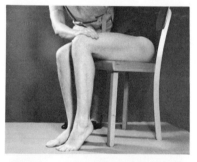

Grades 5b, 4b, 3b
Starting position: Sitting on a chair with the sole of the foot in contact with the floor.
Fixation: Not necessary.
Movement: Plantar flexion by lifting the heel through the full range of movement. The toes must stay on the floor.
Resistance: With the examiner's hand just above the knee. The grades are separated by differences in resistance and the number of repeated movements (three for grade 5, one for grade 4 and one against light resistance for grade 3).

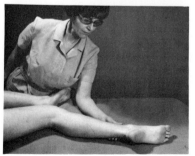

Grade 2
Starting position: Lying on the tested side with flexion at the knee joint and with the foot flexed to 90 degrees and resting on its lateral side. The untested leg rests in front of the body on the plinth and steadies the trunk.
Fixation: The lower leg anteriorly and laterally.
Movement: Plantar flexion through the full range of movement.

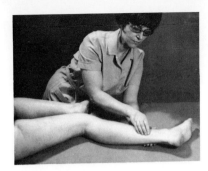

Grades 1, 0

Starting position: Lying on the tested side.

Movement: The Achilles tendon and the soleus (which is situated on the side of the gastrocnemius) can be palpated.

Possible errors

1. If the patient has a tendency to extend the knee joint during the movement, this shows increased activity of the gastrocnemius.
2. Substitution of other muscles (see above).

Shortening

This causes an equinus position of the foot which stays almost the same in both knee extension and knee flexion. In squatting it is not possible to keep the heel on the floor. (Stiffness of the ankle joint must be excluded before the test.)

49 The ankle joint:

Supination with dorsiflexion

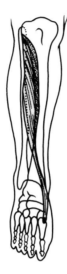

Position of m. tibialis anterior

| | | | L4 | L5 | S1 | | | | | M. tibialis anterior |

General comments

The basic movement is supination and dorsiflexion of the foot.

Grades 5, 4 and 3 are assessed in sitting and grade 2 in lying on the tested side. Grades 1 and 0 are tested supine. The knee joint must be flexed to achieve relaxation of the gastrocnemius. A stretched triceps surae can prevent a full range of movement. The lower leg must be fixed.

Resistance is best given by grasping the foot from underneath with the fingers on its medial side. The resistance is mainly directed towards the base of the first metatarsal bone.

The range of movement is limited by the peronei, the contact between the tarsal bones and the collateral ligament at the lateral malleolus.

Table 49.1

Prime mover	Origin	Insertion	Innervation
Tibialis anterior	Lateral condyle of tibia, proximal two-thirds of lateral surface of tibia and adjoining interosseous membrane	Medial surface of first cuneiform bone, base of first metatarsal (plantar surface)	Deep peroneal nerve L4 L5 (S1)

Assisting muscles: Extensor hallucis longus; extensor digitorum longus in the outer part of the movement
Neutralizers and stabilizers: These hardly exist

Tests

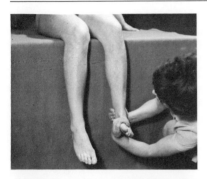

Grades 5, 4
Starting position: Sitting with the lower leg hanging freely, the knee joint in 90 degrees of flexion and the foot in the midposition without touching the floor.
Fixation: The distal third of the lower leg is grasped from behind above the ankle joint without pressure on the tibialis anterior.
Movement: Simultaneous supination and dorsiflexion of the foot. The muscles of the toes must be relaxed.
Resistance: The examiner's fingers are kept against the medial part of the foot to resist abduction and plantar flexion.

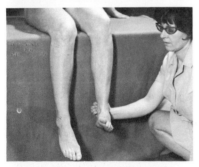

Grade 3
Starting position: Sitting with the lower leg hanging freely over the edge of the plinth. The foot is in the midposition.
Fixation: Above the ankle joint from the dorsal side.
Movement: Supination with dorsiflexion of the foot. The muscles of the toes must be relaxed.

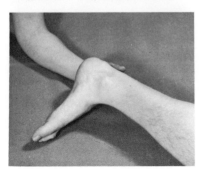

Grade 2
Starting position: Lying on the tested side with semiflexion in the hip and knee joints and the lateral edge of the foot resting on the plinth. The heel is elevated (see Fixation).
Fixation: The distal third of the lower leg from the dorsal side. The heel is lifted lightly and passively so that the edge of the foot rests with the base of the metatarsal against the plinth.
Movement: The patient presses the toes against the plinth and at the same time supinates and dorsiflexes the foot.

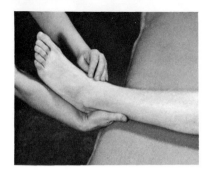

Grades 1, 0

Starting position: Supine lying. The foot is in the midposition with the heel beyond the edge of the plinth.

Fixation: The distal third of the calf. The lateral part of the foot rests on the forearm of the examiner.

Movement: Contraction is palpated on the tendon of the tibialis anterior on the medial part of the foot, above the insertion of the muscle on the base of the first metatarsal or on the line of the tendon over the ankle joint.

Possible errors

1. The lower leg is not fixed above the ankle joint.
2. Grades 1 and 0 are tested without the heel being completely free and beyond the edge of the plinth.
3. Resistance is only given at 90 degrees to the foot and not directly against the direction of movement.
4. If the muscles of the toes are not relaxed, especially the extensor hallucis longus, they may not only help the tibialis anterior but also substitute for its function to a great extent.
5. The necessary flexion in the knee joint to relax the gastrocnemius is omitted.

Shortening

With shortening there is a tendency to a calcaneovarus position of the foot.

50 The ankle joint:

Supination with plantar flexion

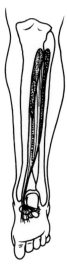

Position of m. tibialis posterior

| | | L4 | L5 | S1 | S2 | | | M. tibialis posterior |

General comments

The basic movement is supination in plantar flexion.

Grades 5, 4 and 3 are tested in lying on the side of the leg to be tested. Grades 2, 1 and 0 are tested in supine lying with the heel beyond the edge of the plinth.

The point of application of resistance is very important. Preferably the fingers should be hung over the inside edge of the foot just behind the metatarsophalangeal joint of the big toe. The direction of resistance is such that the foot would be moved into pronation while at the same time retaining plantar flexion.

The toes should be completely relaxed during the movement. If they strongly flex, this means that substitution of the flexor hallucis longus and flexor digitorum longus is occurring. The range of movement is limited by the peronei, the collateral ligaments, the lateral malleolus and the contact of the tarsal bones.

197

Table 50.1

Prime mover	Origin	Insertion	Innervation
Tibialis posterior	Middle third of the interosseous membrane and adjoining surfaces of tibia and fibula	Tuberosity of the navicular bone, fibrous expansions to the plantar surface of most tarsals and metatarsals	Tibial nerve (L4) L5 S1 (S2)

Assisting muscles: Gastrocnemius, soleus, flexor hallucis longus, flexor digitorum longus
Neutralizers and stabilizers: Hardly exist

Tests

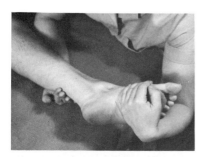

Grades 5, 4
Starting position: Lying on the side of the tested leg with the knee joint flexed.
Fixation: The distal third of the lower leg and the ankle joint are grasped from below.
Movement: Supination of the foot in plantar flexion through the full range of movement. The toes must remain relaxed during the movement.
Resistance: Through the fingers on the medial edge of the foot against the direction of movement.

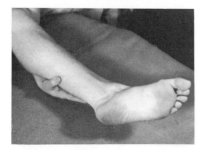

Grade 3
Starting position: Side lying on the side of the leg to be tested with flexion of the knee joint. The foot rests in plantar flexion with its outside edge against the plinth.
Fixation: The distal third of the lower leg on the outside above the ankle joint.
Movement: Supination of the plantar flexed foot.

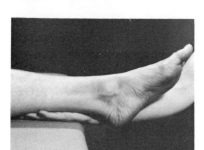

Grade 2
Starting position: Supine lying with the foot plantar flexed and the heel beyond the edge of the plinth.
Fixation: The lower third of the calf from the dorsal side above the ankle.
Movement: Supination of the plantar flexed foot.

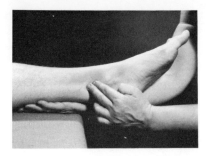

Grades 1, 0
Starting position: Supine lying with the foot plantar flexed and the heel over the edge of the plinth.
Fixation: The lower third of the calf above the ankle.
Movement: The muscle contraction is palpated between the medial malleolus and the navicular bone, and also above and behind the medial malleolus.

Possible errors

1. The test is not valid if grades 2, 1 and 0 are not tested with the heel free beyond the edge of the plinth.
2. When movement is taking place plantar flexion of the foot may not be performed properly.
3. Fixation may not be applied.
4. Mistakes result if resistance is not given in dorsiflexion and abduction at the same time and is separated into its different components.
5. Grades 5, 4 and 3 may not be tested with knee flexion.

Shortening

With this there is a tendency towards the equinovarus position of the foot.

51 The ankle joint:

Plantar pronation

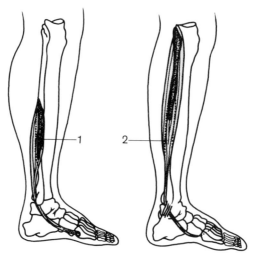

Position of the muscles producing plantar pronation in the ankle joint
(1) m. peroneus brevis, (2) m. peroneus longus

			L4	L5	S1	S2				M. peroneus (fibularis) brevis
			L4	L5	S1	S2				M. peroneus (fibularis) longus

General comments

The basic movement is plantar pronation, that is pronation of the foot from a starting position of plantar flexion.

Grades 5, 4 and 3 are tested in lying on the side of the tested leg or supine with the hip joint medially rotated. Grades 2, 1 and 0 are tested in a supine position with the heel beyond the edge of the plinth.

The muscles of the toes must not take part but stay relaxed during the whole movement. The application of resistance is of great importance: the examiner grasps with the fingers the outside edge of the foot of the leg to be tested and applies resistance to the 'arch' against the direction of the movement.

Sometimes there is an attempt to test the peroneus longus and peroneus brevis separately. Their function is, however, practically the same as is the direction of their muscle fibres and their innervation. Therefore it is possible to separate them only in exceptional cases.

The range of movement is limited by contact between the tarsal bones, the collateral ligament at the medial malleolus and stretching of the tibialis anterior and tibialis posterior.

Table 51.1

Prime mover	Origin	Insertion	Innervation
Peroneus brevis	Distal part of the lateral surface of the fibula	Tuberosity of the fifth metatarsal	Superficial peroneal nerve (L4) L5 S1 (S2)
Peroneus longus	Head of the fibula, lateral condyle of the tibia, proximal half of the lateral surface of the fibula, fascia cruris	Medial cuneiform bone, first metatarsal, occasionally second metatarsal on the plantar surface	Superficial peroneal nerve (L4) L5 S1 (S2)

Assisting muscles: Extensor digitorum longus, peroneus tertius (fifth tendon of the extensor digitorum longus which inserts on the tuberosity of the fifth metatarsal)
Neutralizers and stabilizers: Hardly exist

Tests

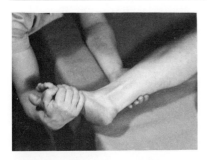

Grades 5, 4
Starting position: Lying on the side of the leg not to be tested with the knee bent. The leg to be tested has the plantar flexed foot resting on the plinth. The toes are relaxed.
Movement: Pronation in plantar flexion through the full range of movement.
Resistance: Against the outside edge of the foot above the fifth metatarsal against the direction of movement.

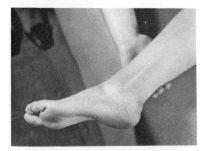

Grade 3
Starting position: Lying on the leg not to be tested and with the leg to be tested steadied against the medial part of the foot and the foot in plantar flexion.
Fixation: The distal third of the lower leg from the medial side.
Movement: Pronation of the foot in plantar flexion.

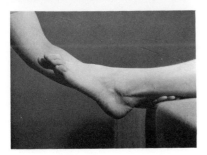

Grade 2
Starting position: Supine lying, with the foot plantar flexed and the heel beyond the edge of the plinth.
Fixation: The distal third of the lower leg.
Movement: Pronation of the plantar-flexed foot through the full range of movement.

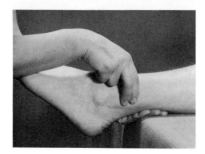

Grades 1, 0

Starting position: Supine lying with the foot plantar flexed and the heel beyond the edge of the plinth.

Fixation: The distal third of the lower leg.

Movement: A slight contraction can be palpated proximally on the tendons on the base of the fifth metatarsal bone and on the outside edge of the lateral malleolus.

Possible errors

1. If fixation of the lower leg is not carried out this is a very important error, especially in children.
2. The starting position of the foot in plantar flexion may not be properly supervised.
3. If the toe muscles are not relaxed during the whole movement the extensor digitorum longus can aid the movement, especially if the peroneus longus is weakened.

Shortening

With shortening there is a tendency to a valgus position of the foot.

52 The metatarsophalangeal joints of the toes:

Flexion

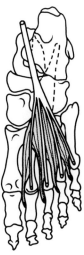

Position of mm. lumbricales

			L5	**S1**	**S2**				M. lumbricalis I
			L5	**S1**	**S2**	S3			Mm. lumbricales II, III, IV

General comments

The basic movement is flexion in the metatarsophalangeal joints of the toes with a movement range of 20–35 degrees.

The foot must always stay in the midposition. Fixation is not always necessary to ensure that the movement really does take place in the main joints. Grades 3 and 2 are not differentiated because the weight of the toes is so small that the movement against gravity has practically no importance.

The range of movement is limited mainly by the toe extensors and also by the contact between the plantar side of the toes and the soft tissue of the foot.

Table 52.1

Prime mover	Origin	Insertion	Innervation
Lumbricales (four) I–IV	Tendons of flexor digitorum longus	Into the extensor tendon connected by fascia with the base of the proximal phalanx and the capsule of the joint	I: medial plantar nerve L5 S1 (S2) II–IV: Lateral plantar nerve L5 S1 S2 S3

Table 52.2

Prime mover	Origin	Insertion	Innervation
Flexor hallucis brevis	Medial, intermedial and lateral cuneiform bones (plantar surface) and the navicular bone	Medial head: unites with the tendon of abductor hallucis and inserts into the medial sesamoid bone of the hallux Lateral head: unites with the tendon of adductor hallucis and inserts into the lateral sesamoid bone of the hallux	Medial head: medial plantar nerve L5 S1 Lateral head: lateral plantar nerve S1 S2

Tests

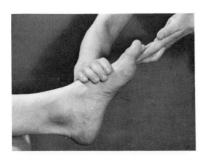

Grades 5, 4
Starting position: Supine lying or sitting. The leg to be tested is extended at the hip and knee joints. The foot is in the midposition.
Fixation: The foot is grasped in such a way that the thumb is underneath the metatarsal heads.
Movement: Flexion in the metatarsophalangeal joints of the second to fifth toes.
Resistance: With the fingers against the proximal metatarsophalangeal joint from the plantar side.

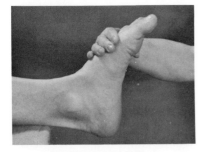

Grades 3–2
Starting position: Supine lying or sitting with the leg to be tested outstretched and the foot in the midposition.
Fixation: With the thumb under the metatarsal head.
Movement: Flexion of the proximal phalanx, possibly without flexion of the big toe.

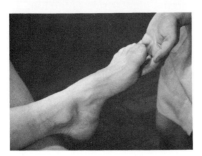

Grades 1, 0
Palpation is usually useless. It is better to observe the movement of the toes.

Possible errors

1. Fixation of the metatarsal bones may be omitted.
2. The movement may not take place in the metatarso-phalangeal joints and the other phalangeal joints may move.
3. During the movement the correct position of the foot may not be controlled.
4. If the lumbricales are weakened, substitution by the long toe flexor occurs. This can be noted through hyperextension in the metatarsophalangeal joints and flexion in the inter-phalangeal joints.

Shortening

This results in a flexion position and decreased extension in the metatarsophalangeal joints.

53 The metatarsophalangeal joint of the hallux:

Flexion

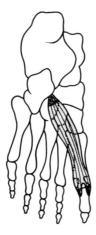

Position of m. flexor hallucis brevis

| | | | **L5** | **S1** | **S2** | | | M. flexor hallucis brevis

General comments

The basic movement is flexion of the metatarsophalangeal joint of the hallux through a range of 20–30 degrees.

The foot must always be in the midposition. Fixation is not always necessary. Grades 3 and 2 are not differentiated because the weight of the big toe is too small.

The range of movement is limited mainly by the dorsal part of the joint capsule and the extensors of the big toe.

Table 53.1

Prime mover	Origin	Insertion	Innervation
M. flexor hallucis brevis	Flat surface of the first, intermediate and lateral cuneiform bones and the navicular bone	Medial-head: merging with the M. abductor hallucis tendon and inserting on the medial joint of the hallux	Medial-head: N. plantaris medialis L5 S1
		Lateral head merging with the M. abductor hallucis tendon and inserting on the lateral joint of the hallux	Lateral head: N. plantaris lateralis S1 S2

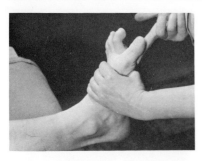

Grades 5, 4
Starting position: Supine lying or sitting with the leg to be tested held in a straight position at the knee and hip joints with the foot in the midposition.
Fixation: The first metatarsal by gripping its head.
Movement: Flexion of the proximal phalanx of the big toe at the main joint through the full range of movement. Motion of the other toes cannot usually be excluded.
Resistance: One finger against the plantar side of the proximal phalanx of the big toe.

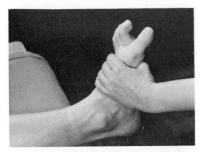

Grades 3, 2
Starting position, fixation and movement: The same as for grades 5 and 4.
Resistance: Not given.

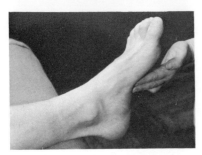

Grades 1, 0
Movement: A flicker is observed in the big toe in the direction of flexion and the flexor hallucis brevis is palpated on the inside edge of the sole of the foot.

Possible errors

1. The movement may not take place only in the main joint.
2. The foot may not be kept in the midposition.

Shortening

This results in a flexion position and decreased extension in the metatarsophalangeal joint of the hallux.

54 The metatarsophalangeal joints of the toes:

Extension

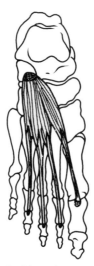

Position of m. extensor digitorum brevis

			L4	L5	S1	S2				M. extensor digitorum longus
			L4	L5	S1	S2				M. extensor digitorum brevis
			L4	L5	S1					M. extensor hallucis brevis

General comments

The basic movement is extension in the metatarsophalangeal joints of the toes over a range of 80 degrees.

All the tests are performed supine.

It is very important for the foot to stay in the midposition. If there is pronounced plantar flexion of the foot, the extensors are stretched. If there is excessive dorsiflexion the muscles are relaxed and cannot show their full strength. Grades 3 and 2 can be differentiated because of the slight weight of the toes.

Four extensors are involved in extension of the toes, namely two for the big toe and two for the other toes.

The extensor digitorum longus extends the second to fifth toes but the extensor digitorum brevis has no tendon for the little toe. Because of this they can be differentiated. If the patient can move only the second to fourth toes this means that the function of the long toe extensor is diminished or abolished.

Palpation of the muscle contraction is a further aid to differential diagnosis.

Fixation of the foot is necessary to retain the midposition.

The big toe and the other toes must be examined separately. In practice this is not always possible because not everyone can extend the four lateral toes without moving the big toe. Therefore all the toes are usually tested together, although resistance is applied separately to the big toe and to the other toes.

The range of movement is limited mainly by the plantar ligaments and the flexors.

Table 54.1

Prime mover	Origin	Insertion	Innervation
Extensor digitorum longus	Lateral condyle of the tibia, proximal half of the medial surface of the fibula, adjacent parts of the interosseous membrane	Divides into four tendons to the second to fifth toes, the tendons are attached to the dorsal expansion which inserts into the terminal phalanges	Deep peroneal nerve L4 L5 S1 (S2)
Extensor digitorum brevis	Upper surface of the calcaneus	Divides into three thin tendons for the second to fourth toes; inserts with extensor digitorum longus into the dorsal expansion	Deep peroneal nerve (L4) L5 S1 (S2)
Extensor hallucis brevis	Upper surface of the calcaneus (medially to extensor digitorum brevis)	Proximal phalanx of hallux and the dorsal expansion	Deep peroneal nerve L4 L5 S1

Tests

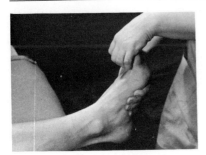

Grades 5, 4

Starting position: Supine lying or sitting with the foot in the midposition.

Fixation: All the metatarsal bones by gripping around the foot from the plantar side.

Movement: Extension of the proximal toes.

Resistance: Against the dorsum of the proximal phalanx.

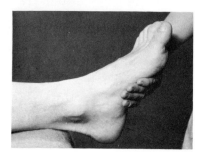

Grades 3–2
Starting position: Supine lying, with the foot in the midposition.
Fixation: The foot from the plantar side.
Movement: Extension of the toes in the proximal joint.

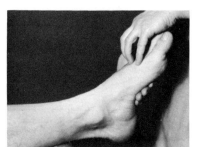

Grades 1, 0
Starting position: The foot in the midposition.
Fixation: Not necessary.
Movement: The tendons of the long extensor are palpated on the dorsum of the metatarsals and the muscle bulk of the short extensor is palpated lateral to the long tendons in front of the lateral malleolus.

Possible errors

1. The foot may not be in the midposition through the full range of movement.
2. The short and long extensors may not be properly differentiated.

Shortening

Hyperextension in the proximal joints of the toes causes a secondary flexion position of the interphalangeal joints.

55 The metatarsophalangeal joints of the toes:

Adduction

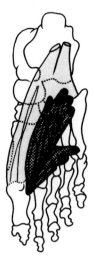

Position of m. adductor hallucis

| | | | | | S1 | S2 | S3 | | Mm. interossei plantares |
| | | | | | S1 | S2 | S3 | | M. adductor hallucis |

General comments

The basic movement is adduction of the toes from a starting position of maximal abduction.

The range of movement is dependent on the starting position and the abduction varies between 10 and 20 degrees. Examination takes place supine or sitting with the foot in the midposition. The muscle strength varies even in the normal foot and therefore it is best to compare the movement with that in the other foot when testing. In man this movement is practically without functional importance.

The range of movement is limited by contact between the toes.

Table 55.1

Prime mover	Origin	Insertion	Innervation
Dorsal interossei	Medial sides of the third, fourth and fifth metatarsals	Medial side of the proximal phalanges of the third–fifth toes, and the dorsal digital expansions	Lateral plantar nerve S1 S2 (S3)
Abductor hallucis	Oblique head: cuboid bone, lateral cuneiform bone, plantar ligament, second and fourth metatarsals. Transverse head: plantar surface of the proximal joint of the fourth and often also the fifth toe	Medial side of the proximal phalanx of the hallux with the tendon of flexor hallucis brevis (lateral muscle bulk)	Lateral plantar nerve S1 S2 (S3)

Tests

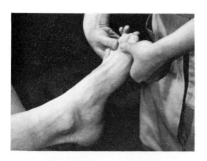

Grades 5, 4
Starting position: Supine lying or sitting with the leg extended at the knee joint and the foot in the midposition.
Fixation: The examiner holds the toes in abduction.
Movement: Adduction of the toes.
Resistance: Against the proximal phalanges of the toes from the second toe outwards against both sides.

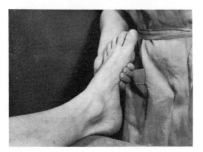

Grades 3, 2, 1, 0
One can only establish whether the patient can perform the movement. One must not forget that the toes must spontaneously return to their starting position from abduction.

Possible errors

These hardly ever occur.

Shortening

This is manifested by difficulty in achieving abduction, even passively. Adduction position of the big toe results.

212

56 The metatarsophalangeal joints of the toes:

Abduction

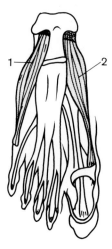

Abduction muscles in the metatarsophalangeal joints of the toes
(1) m. abductor digiti minimi, (2) m. abductor hallucis

				S1	S2	S3		Mm. interossei dorsales
			L5	S1				M. abductor hallucis
			L5	S1	S2	S3		M. abductor digiti minimi

General comments

The basic movement is abduction of the toes over a range of 10–20 degrees.

During the test the foot must be in the midposition. In man this movement is of hardly any functional significance and its strength is very varied even in the normal foot. To get a good result the other foot must also be tested. Usually it is only possible to ascertain whether the movement can be performed.

The range of movement is limited by the collateral ligaments of the toe joints and the stretching of the skin between the toes.

Table 56.1

Prime mover	Origin	Insertion	Innervation
Dorsal interossei	Each muscle: two heads from adjacent sides of the metatarsals between which it lies	Proximal phalanx: lateral side of the second toe second—fourth proximal phalanges: the second toe has two dorsal interossei	Lateral plantar nerve S1 S2 (S3)
Abductor hallucis	Medial process of the tuberosity of the calcaneus	Medial side of the first phalanx of the hallux	Medial plantar nerve L5 S1
Abductor digiti minimi	Lateral process of the tuberosity of the calcaneus	Lateral side of the first phalanx of the hallux	Lateral plantar nerve (L5) S1 S2 (S3)

Tests

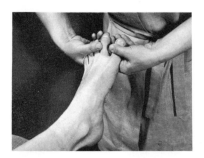

Grades 5, 4
Starting position: Supine lying or sitting with the knee in extension and the foot in the midposition.
Fixation: Not necessary.
Movement: Abduction of the toes through the full range of movement.
Resistance: Mainly against the medial inside edge of the big toe and thereafter against the outside of the third to fifth toes and the inside and outside of the second toe.

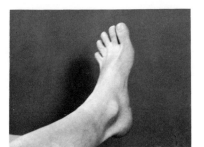

Grades 3—2
Starting position and movement: As for grades 5 and 4.
Resistance: Not given.

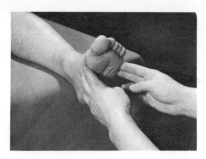

Grades 1, 0

Movement: The abductor hallucis and abductor minimi are palpable over the medial and lateral edges of the foot.

Possible errors

Errors hardly ever occur.

Shortening

This is very pronounced, especially in the big toe in which a position of abduction results.

215

57 The proximal interphalangeal joints of the toes:

Flexion

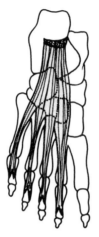

Position of m. flexor digitorum brevis

| | | | **L5** | **S1** | | | | M. flexor digitorum brevis

General comments

The basic movement is flexion in the proximal interphalangeal joints through a range of 70 degrees.

The foot must be in the midposition. If there is plantar flexion, the long extensors are stretched and so the flexion is decreased. In pareses of the gastrocnemius and soleus the heel must be fixed because of the origin of the flexor digitorum brevis. Without fixation the heel moves towards the forefoot, the longitudinal arch of the foot increases and movement is almost impossible.

Grades 3 and 2 are not differentiated.

Table 57.1

Prime mover	Origin	Insertion	Innervation
Flexor digitorum brevis	Medial process of the tuberosity of the calcaneus; plantar aponeurosis	Two slips into sides of the second phalanges of the lateral four toes	Medial plantar nerve L5 S1

Assisting muscles: Flexor digitorum longus, quadratus plantae

Table 57.2

Prime mover	Origin	Insertion	Innervation
Flexor digitorum longus	Posterior surface of the middle third of the tibia	Distal phalanges of the lateral four toes	Tibial nerve L5 S1 (S2)

Assisting muscle: Quadratus plantae

Tests

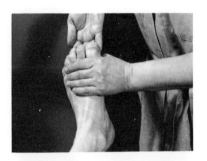

Grades 5, 4
Starting position: Supine lying or sitting with the foot in the midposition.
Fixation: The proximal phalanges of the toes with the thumb on the plantar side and the fingers on the dorsum.
Movement: Flexion of the second to fifth toes in the proximal interphalangeal joints.
Resistance: Against the plantar side of the middle phalanges of the second to fifth toes. (For the fourth and fifth toes this is more or less impossible because of the very short phalanges.)

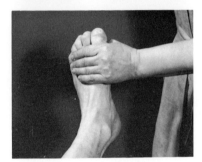

Grades 3–2
Starting position, fixation and movement: As above.
Resistance: Not given.

Grades 1, 0
Movement: A jerk in the toes is observed. The tendons cannot be easily palpated.

Possible errors

1. If the gastrocnemius and soleus are shortened the test must not take place with the knee straight.
2. When the gastrocnemius and soleus are paralysed, fixation of the heel is important.
3. The midposition of the foot may not be retained.

Shortening

This results in a flexion position with decreased dorsal flexion in the proximal interphalangeal joints.

217

58 The distal interphalangeal joints of the toes:

Flexion

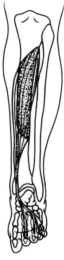

Position of m. flexor digitorum longus

| | | | **L5** | **S1** | **S2** | | | | M. flexor digitorum longus |

General comments

The basic movement is flexion in the distal interphalangeal joints through a range of about 50 degrees. If the gastrocnemius and soleus are shortened, the leg must be flexed at the knee joint to maintain the midposition of the foot. The flexor digitorum longus is a long muscle which passes behind the medial malleolus. With plantar flexion of the foot this muscle is relaxed and cannot utilize its full strength. At the same time the extensors are stretched, thus increasing the resistance.

Table 58.1

Prime mover	Origin	Insertion	Innervation
Flexor digitorum longus	Mid-third of the dorsal side of the tibia	End joint of the second to fifth toes	N. tibialis L5 S1 (S2)

Assisting muscles: Quadratus plantae

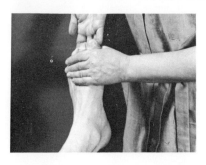

Grades 5, 4
Starting position: Supine lying or sitting with the foot in the midposition.
Fixation: The middle phalanges of the toes are held with the thumb from the plantar side. The other fingers grip the foot and the phalanges of the toes from the dorsum.
Movement: Flexion of the second to fifth toes in the distal interphalangeal joints. Because of the shortness of the fourth and fifth toes, separation between them is not possible.
Resistance: Against the distal phalanges of the second to fifth toes.

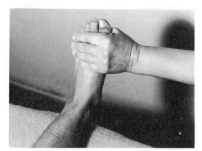

Grades 3–2
Starting position, fixation and movement: As grades 5 and 4.
Resistance: Not given.

Grades 1, 0
Movement: A jerk of the toes can be observed.

Possible errors

The midposition of the foot may not be maintained. Flexion in the knee joint is necessary if there is a contracture of the gastrocnemius and soleus.

Shortening

This causes a flexion position of the second to fifth toes in the interphalangeal and metatarsophalangeal joints. Decreased extension and slight pronation of the foot are observed.

59 The interphalangeal joint of the hallux:

Flexion

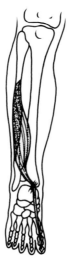

Position of m. flexor hallucis longus

| | | | | **L5** | **S1** | **S2** | | | | M. flexor hallucis longus

General comments

The basic movement is flexion in the interphalangeal joint of the big toe through a range of 70 degrees.

The foot must stay in the midposition. In pronounced plantar flexion the muscle is excessively relaxed and at the same time there is stretching of the extensors. The metatarsophalangeal joint must be fixed because evaluation of the long flexors is impossible if the short flexor is overactive.

Grades 3 and 2 are not differentiated.

Table 59.1

Prime mover	Origin	Insertion	Innervation
Flexor hallucis longus	Distal two thirds of posterior surface of fibula and adjacent interosseus membrane	Distal phalanx of the hallux	Tibial nerve L5 S1 S2

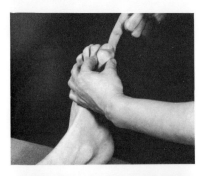

Grades 5, 4
Starting position: Supine lying or sitting with the foot in the midposition.
Fixation: The proximal phalanx of the big toe from both sides so that the proximal joint is slightly extended.
Movement: Flexion in the interphalangeal joint of the hallux.
Resistance: Against the plantar side of the distal phalanx of the toe.

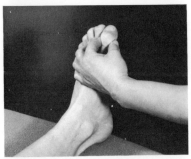

Grades 3, 2
Starting position: Supine lying or sitting with the foot in the midposition.
Fixation: The proximal phalanx of the big toe from both sides.
Movement: Flexion in the interphalangeal joint of the hallux.

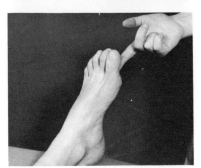

Grades 1, 0
Movement: Increased tension in the tendon can be palpated on the plantar side of the proximal phalanx of the big toe. Better, a jerk may be seen in the distal phalanx.

Possible errors

1. The proximal phalanx may not be fixed.

Shortening

This causes a flexion position of the big toe.

60　The interphalangeal joint of the hallux:

Extension

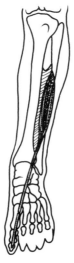

Position of m. extensor hallucis longus

| | | |L4 |L5 |S1 |S2 | | | | M. extensor hallucis longus

General comments

The basic movement is extension in the interphalangeal joint through a range of 80 degrees (from maximal flexion).

All tests take place with the patient supine. The foot must be in the midposition to give the best conditions for movement.

Grades 3 and 2 are not differentiated because of the low weight of the toes.

Fixation is necessary to keep the foot in the correct position.

The range of movement is limited mainly by the plantar part of the joint capsule and flexor hallucis longus.

Table 60.1

Prime mover	Origin	Insertion	Innervation
Extensor hallucis longus	Middle part of anterior surface of fibula and interosseous membrane	Dorsal surface of the distal phalanx of the hallux	Deep peroneal nerve (L4) L5 S1 (S2)

222

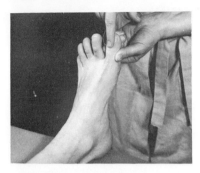

Grades 5, 4
Starting position: Supine lying or sitting with the foot in the exact midposition.
Fixation: The proximal phalanx of the big toe from both sides.
Movement: Extension in the interphalangeal joint of the hallux through the full range.
Resistance: Against the dorsal side of the distal phalanx of the hallux (against the nail of the toe).

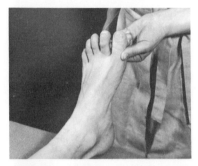

Grades 3–2
Starting position: Supine lying or sitting with the foot in the midposition.
Fixation: The proximal phalanx.
Movement: Extension in the interphalangeal joint of the hallux.

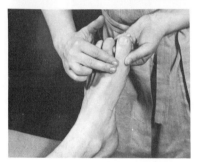

Grades 1, 0
Movement: A trace of contraction or a jerk can be palpated at the tendon above the proximal joint.

Possible errors

1.   The foot may not be in the midposition.

Shortening

This causes hyperextension of the big toe.

Section 2 Assessment of the most common shortened muscle groups

The meanings of the words contracture, shortening, muscle tightness and muscle tone are often the subject of confusion. This applies especially to the first term, as physiologists, orthopaedic

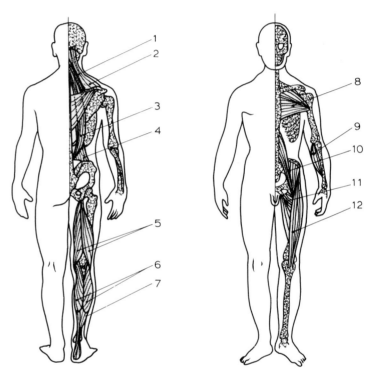

Rear view
(1) m. levator scapulae (under), (2) m. trapezius (upper portion), (3) m. erector spinae, (4) m. quadratus lumborum, (5) knee joint muscle group, (6) m. gastrocnemius, (7) m. soleus
Front view
(8) m. pectoralis major, (9) hand and finger flexors, (10) m. iliopsoas, (11) adductors of the thigh, (12) m. rectus femoris

surgeons, neurologists, rheumatologists, physiatrists and physiotherapists often have different meanings for the same expressions.

According to physiologists, a muscle contracture is a reflex condition, often provoked by pain. It may show irregular electromyographic activity.

To orthopaedic surgeons, a contracture is a change in the muscles and connective tissue of other soft joint structures. It can take place after peripheral paresis and is sometimes associated with a change in the structure of the muscle. Such a contracture does not produce any EMG activity.

From a neurologist's view a contracture is usually a painful reflex condition, as for example, in acute low back pain. This corresponds to the physiological view of contracture. Neurologists also refer to another type of contracture in which there is a change in the connective tissue of the muscle, such as in peripheral paresis (see above). A patient who has spasticity shows a completely different type of contracture, as a result of the increase in stretch reflex. Another type of contracture is of ischaemic origin, as in Volkmann's ischaemia. Patients with a poor posture very often develop shortened or contracted muscles for unknown reasons. In these cases it is not clear to what extent the muscle fibres or connective tissues are involved. The type of shortening discussed in this book falls into the last mentioned category and corresponds most closely to the concept of muscle tightness. It is evident that there are many different reasons for a muscle to become shortened (meaning that the muscle is shorter than normal, even at rest). Shortened muscles cannot allow a full range of movement in the joint, either through contraction of the antagonist muscle or through passive stretching. Muscle shortening does not show any spontaneous electrical activity and therefore does not involve active muscle contraction or increased activity in the nervous system. Shortening can take place through a change in the relative strengths of antagonistic muscle groups, as in poliomyelitis, or after injury to the nerve.

Some muscle groups react in a relatively stereotyped manner in different pathological situations, for example, with shortening or with weakening. To date, muscle shortening has not been described in sufficient detail, even though its influence on affected muscles can be of great importance in the pathology of altered movement. An understanding of these shortened muscles and their behaviour is especially useful in the treatment of muscles with no paresis.

A tendency of muscle shortening is noticeable not only during illness, but also as an apparently typical reaction by some muscle groups even in normal circumstances. The muscles of postural importance show the greatest tendency to shorten. These muscles in man are those that make standing possible, and above all standing on one leg. This is the most common postural position for man; for instance, 85 per cent of the walking cycle is spent standing on one leg. Those muscles with a postural function are genetically older and demonstrate less reaction to different injuries. They have different physiological and probably also biochemical qualities to muscles with a mainly phasic function. The latter normally weaken and exhibit signs of inhibition.

The assessment of shortened muscle groups must be as exact as a muscle function test for a weakened muscle, and the same standardized routine must be maintained. As it is difficult to determine the exact grade of many muscles, a general estimate is considered sufficient. Where it is possible to measure the angle between two extremities the assessment of shortened muscles can be very accurate. To obtain a reliable evaluation the starting position, method of fixation and direction of movement must be observed extremely carefully. As in muscle function testing the prime mover must not be exposed to external pressure.

If possible, the force exerted on the tested muscle must not work over two joints. The examiner performs at an even speed a slow movement that brakes slowly at the end of the range. To keep the stretch and the muscle irritability about equal the movement must not be jerky. Pressure or pull must always act in the required direction of movement. Muscle shortening can only be correctly evaluated if the joint range is not decreased as is a bony limitation or joint restriction.

Muscles with mainly postural function

Sternocleidomastoid
Pectoralis major (clavicular and sternal end)
Trapezius (upper part)
Levator scapulae
Flexors of the upper extremity

Quadratus lumborum

Back extensors
   Erector spinae
   Longissimus thoracis
   Rotatores
   Multifidus

Hip flexors
   Iliopsoas
   Tensor fasciae latae
   Rectus femoris

Lateral rotators of the hip
   Piriformis

Medial rotators of the hip
   Pectineus
   Adductor longus
   Adductor brevis
   Adductor magnus

Hamstrings
   Biceps femoris
   Semitendinosus
   Semimembranosus

Plantar flexors
   Gastrocnemius
   Soleus
   Tibialis posterior

Muscles with mainly dynamic (phasic) function
Scaleni
Pectoralis major (abdominal part)
Subscapularis
Extensors of the upper extremity
Trapezius (lower part)
Rhomboidei
Serratus anterior
Rectus abdominis
Obliquus abdominis externus, obliquus abdominis internus
Gluteus minimus, gluteus medius, gluteus maximus
Vastus medialis and lateralis
Tibalis anterior
Peronei

61 Gastrocnemius and soleus

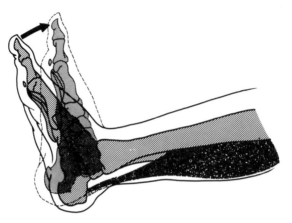

The gastrocnemius and soleus muscles

Tests

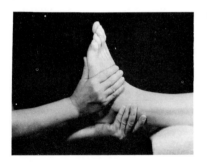

Gastrosoleus

Starting position: Supine lying with both legs outstretched and the heels outside the examination plinth.

Grasp: The right hand of the examiner grasps the right Achilles tendon just above the heel without causing pressure on the tendons (when examining the left leg the examiner uses the left hand). The fingers are outstretched and the lower arm is held as a prolongation of the lower leg. The other hand is placed on the outside edge of the foot with the fingers on the dorsum of the foot and the thumb on the sole parallel with the outside edge.

Fixation: Not necessary.

Stretch: The main stretch is applied to the heel distally in the direction of the muscle fibres. The thumb of the other hand steers the forefoot with a light perpendicular pressure to prevent sideways movement of the foot.

Range of movement: Flexion to 90 degrees should be achieved without difficulty.

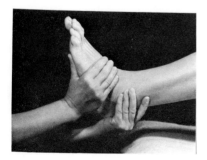

Soleus

The assessment is the same but the knee joint should be passively flexed to exclude gastrocnemius activity.

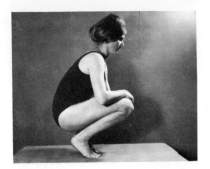

An orientation test for the soleus

The patient crouches with slight forward flexion of the trunk. The knees should be parallel to, but not touching each other. If the range of movement in the joint is not restricted, the patient should be able to squat with the heels on the floor.

Possible errors

1. If the examiner's thumb is not on top of and parallel with the outside edge of the foot but more towards the middle of the sole of the foot, then a reflex reaction of the gastrocnemius and soleus will result.
2. If the thumb does not press along the whole of its length, but only close to its tip, then the direction of the movement is altered and different structures are stimulated (in particular the plantar aponeurosis and quadratus plantae).
3. When pressure is applied incorrectly to the dorsum of the forefoot and the necessary strong stretch of the heel does not take place, the muscles in the sole of the foot but not the gastrocnemius and soleus are caused to stretch.
4. If the forearm is not held as a prolongation of the lower leg the direction of the stretch is changed.
5. The leg may not be stationary on the plinth but may be lifted upwards.

62 The hip flexors:

Iliopsoas, rectus femoris, tensor fasciae latae and short adductors

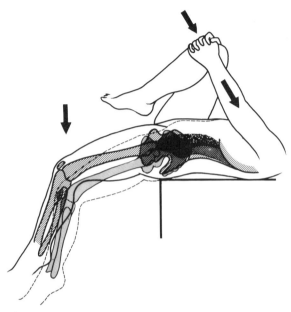

Flexors of the hip joint
m. iliopsoas, m. rectus femoris, m. tensor fasciae latae and thigh shortening adductors

Tests

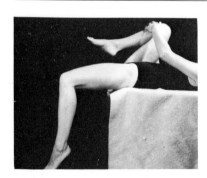

Starting position: Supine lying, with the coccyx just outside the plinth. The passive leg is flexed as far as possible so that the pelvis is tilted backwards and the lumbar lordosis is eliminated. The leg is fixed in this position by holding the fixed knee (a long lever). If this knee flexion is painful it is better to fix the whole knee joint (see picture b).

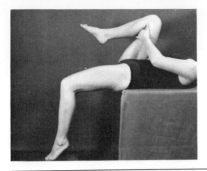

Fixation: Throughout the test the passive leg must be fixed towards the trunk by constant pressure to eliminate the lordosis of the lumbar spine. During the evaluation the examiner pushes the leg further against the trunk.

Normal finding: The thigh is horizontal and the lower leg hangs vertically. The patella is situated slightly lateral to the knee joint. On the outer side of the thigh there is a very slight deepening.

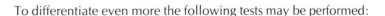

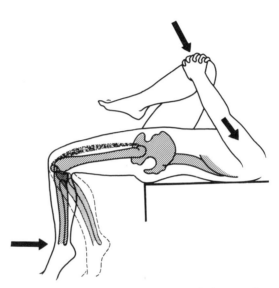

Pathological finding: A flexion position in the hip joint shows shortening of the iliopsoas. The lower leg positioned diagonally downwards indicates that the rectus femoris is shortened. A flexion position of the hip joint with a simultaneous tendency to extension in the knee joint points to shortening of both the iliopsoas and rectus femoris. Lateral deviation of the patella and more pronounced deepening on the outside of the thigh shows on a shortened tensor fasciae latae and iliotibial band.

To differentiate even more the following tests may be performed:

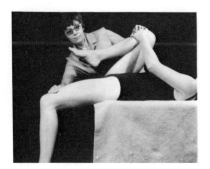

1. Pressure is applied to the lower third of the thigh:
    (i) in the direction of the hyperextension of the hip joint. When extension cannot increase this indicates shortening of the iliopsoas. When there is a simultaneous compensatory extension in the knee joint this points to shortening of the rectus femoris.
    (ii) in the direction of the adduction of the hip joint. Increased deepening on the outside of the thigh over the iliotibial tract shows shortening of the tensor fasciae latae and the iliotibial tract.

231

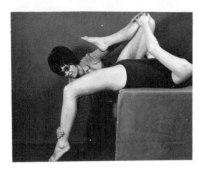

(iii) in the direction of the abduction of the hip joint. The decreased range of movement and compensatory flexion of the hip joint are signs of shortening of the one-joint thigh adductors.

2. Pressure is applied to the lower third of the lower leg to increase knee flexion. If flexion is painful and difficult this shows shortening of the rectus femoris. Further pressure may cause compensatory flexion in the hip joint, simultaneously a deepening appears immediately above the patella. This shows shortening of the rectus femoris.

Orientation tests for the iliopsoas and rectus femoris

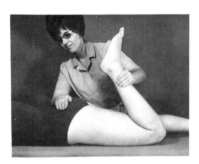

Starting position: Prone with the legs outstretched. If the iliopsoas is shortened the hip joint remains in flexion. Passive flexion in the knee joint provokes a compensatory increase of flexion in the hip joint, and hyperlordosis of the lumbar spine is a sign of shortened rectus femoris. This test is not very sensitive.

An orientation test in standing for the iliopsoas and gastrocnemius and soleus

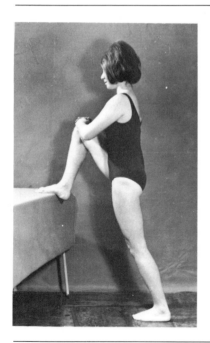

The patient stands as far as possible from the plinth while steadying the leg that is not to be tested against it. The leg to be tested is situated exactly in between medial and lateral rotation. The foot is in the sagittal plane and the sole rests on the floor. The knee is in extension. The position of the sole of the foot and the hip joint is checked for shortening of the gastrocnemius and soleus, and of the iliopsoas respectively. From the standing position the patient shifts the pelvis forwards without rotating it and without increasing the lumbar lordosis. With a shortened gastrocnemius and soleus the heel is lifted from the floor, and with a shortened iliopsoas the hyperextension of 5–10 degrees in the hip joint is not possible. This test is also suitable as a home exercise to stretch these muscles.

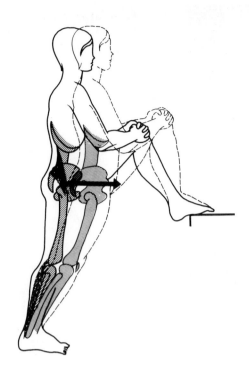

Possible errors

1. Insufficient fixation of the pelvis enables a change of position and increased lordosis of the lumbar spine.
2. The patient is not relaxing sufficiently and the lower leg is knowingly held in slight extension in the knee joint.
3. The direction of the pressure may not be maintained. In particular during examination of a shortened rectus femoris, compensatory flexion in the hip may be supported if pressure is wrongly directed upwards during passive flexion in the knee joint.
4. The movement may be performed too quickly.
5. The muscle groups may not be differentiated.
6. The patient fixes the not tested leg only by himself and no additional fixation may be given.
7. In the orientation test in standing, forward flexion of the trunk or increased lumbar lordosis may be allowed during the movement, together with lateral rotation in the hip joint of the leg to be tested.

63 The hamstrings

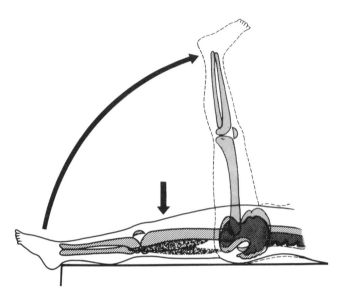

The hamstrings
m. biceps femoris, m. semitendinosus and m. semimembranosus

Tests

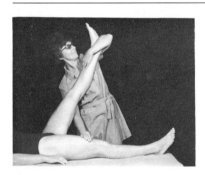

Test when the hip flexors are not shortened

Starting position: Supine lying, with the legs outstretched.
Fixation: The lower third of the thigh on the leg not to be tested without touching the patella.
Grasp: The examiner grasps the lower leg of the patient so that the knee is kept in extension through pressure from above. The heel is held in the crook of the examiner's elbow with the foot against her upper arm to prevent lateral rotation of the leg.
Movement: Flexion in the hip joint.
Normal range of movement: Flexion over a range of about 80 degrees.

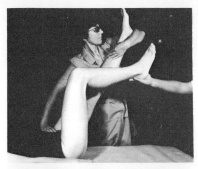

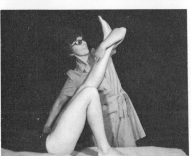

Test when the hip flexors are shortened

Shortening of the hip flexors causes a forward tilt of the pelvis and so the hamstrings are already stretched and the test result cannot be accurate. Therefore, this second modification is necessary for correct examination.

Starting position: Supine, with the leg not to be tested flexed at the hip and knee joints (passively) or (less suitably) flexed with the sole of the foot on the plinth. Thus the lumbar spine is kept flat on the plinth and there is no kyphosis or lordosis of the lumbar spine.
Fixation: The pelvis.
Grasp: As in the previous test.
Range of motion: Flexion to 90 degrees. In comparison to the previous test the range is 10–15 degrees greater.

Possible errors

1. The not tested leg is not fixed.
2. Fixation is given over the knee joint on top of the patella despite the fact that the joint should be free.
3. At examination an increase in flexion is allowed in the knee joint together with abduction and lateral rotation of the hip joint. This can be made even worse if the examiner does not start the movement from her own shoulder joint and if she turns in such a way that abduction is performed by the leg of the patient.
4. If there is shortening of the hip flexors, which is very common, the not tested leg is not put in the flexion position during the test.

235

64 The adductors of the thigh:

Pectineus, adductor brevis, adductor magnus, adductor longus, biceps femoris, semitendinosus, semimembranosus, gracilis

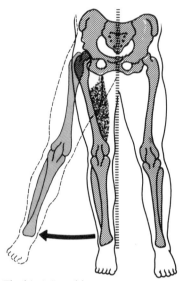

The hip joint adductors
pectineus, adductor brevis, adductor magnus, adductor longus, biceps femoris, semitendinosus, semimembranosus and gracilis

Tests

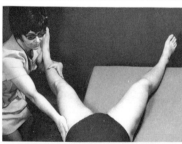

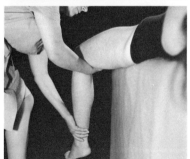

Starting position: Supine lying, with the leg to be tested close to the edge of the plinth. The leg not to be tested is 15–25 degrees abducted in the hip joint with the heel over the edge of the plinth.

Grip: The leg to be tested is placed with the heel in the crook of the examiner's elbow. Her hand is placed on the anterolateral aspect of the tibia, so maintaining the knee in extension through forward pressure on the lower leg. The foot of the patient is steadied on the upper arm of the examiner to prevent lateral rotation in the hip joint.

Fixation: The pelvis or leg not to be tested (as far as possible).

Movement: Abduction of the extended leg in the hip joint over the maximal range. When the full movement is performed the knee joint is passively flexed and abduction continued.

Normal range of movement: Abduction to about 40 degrees with an extended and flexed knee. If the range of movement of the hip joint with the knee extended or flexed is limited to the same or almost the same extent, the one-joint adductors, mainly the pectineus and the adductors, are proved to be shortened. If the range of movement increased with the knee extended is limited and normal with a flexed knee then the two-joint adductors (namely the gracilis, biceps femoris, semimembranosus and semitendinosus) are shortened.

236

Possible errors

1. During abduction there is also some flexion or lateral rotation in the hip joint.
2. The examination does not take place in the two different positions described, that is with an extended and a flexed knee.
3. The necessary slight abduction of the leg not to be tested does not take place and so the fixation of the pelvis is insufficient.
4. The pelvis is not fixed.

65 Piriformis

Tests

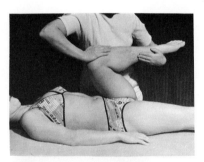

Starting position: Supine, with the leg to be tested flexed at the hip and knee joints.
Fixation: The pelvis through pressure from the examiner's hand against the knee in the direction of the longitudinal axis of the thigh.
Movement: The leg to be tested is flexed, adducted and medially rotated during fixation of the pelvis as above. Medial rotation in the hip joint is possible through pressure against the medial part of the lower leg.

If there is shortening of the piriformis, adduction and medial rotation are decreased and are painful at the end of the range of motion.

Palpation of the piriformis usually gives better results than the stretch test. The palpation is performed deeply in the area of the greater sciatic foramen across the muscle fibres. Normally the muscle is not palpable, but if there is shortening then it is felt and it moves away under the examiner's fingers.

Possible errors

1. Pressure against the knee is not constant during the examination and so the fixation of the pelvis is insufficient.
2. Adduction and medial rotation is not carried out to the end of the range.

66 Quadratus lumborum

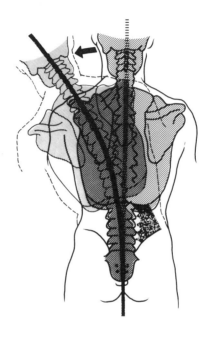

Tests

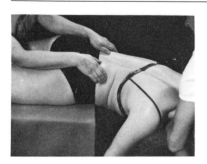

Starting position: Prone lying, with the upper part of the body over the end of the plinth.

Fixation: One examiner fixes the pelvis and the legs, and during the movement palpates the tension of the quadratus lumborum. The other examiner steadies the upper part of the patient's body with her forearm without putting pressure on the throat of the patient.

Movement: Side flexion of the trunk in the horizontal plane without twisting, lowering, or lifting.

Normal range: The side flexion of the trunk should be symmetrical. If there is muscle shortening, the spinal column does not show a smooth arched curve during side flexion, the lumbar spine stays very stiff and there is a compensatory increase of the movement in the thoracolumbar segments.

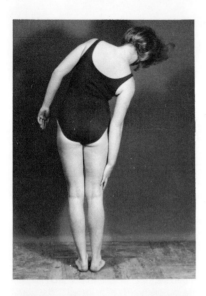

Orientation test in standing

The patient is standing in side flexion without twisting the trunk forwards or backwards or lifting the shoulders. A sideways movement of the pelvis towards the opposite side must be avoided. The range of movement of the two sides is compared.

At the end position, normally the line from the axilla of the opposite shoulder coincides with the intergluteal line. This test is not reliable in standing because the patient cannot be fully relaxed and the tested quadratus lumborum muscle contracts eccentrically during the movement.

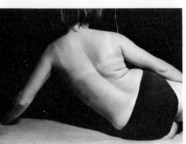

Orientation test in side lying

The patient lies on the side to be examined with the leg slightly flexed to stabilize the body. The top arm rests on the body and the bottom one is slightly flexed at the elbow with the hand resting on the plinth above the head.
Fixation: Not necessary.
Movement: The patient pushes on her lower arm and therefore slowly raises her body. Thus side flexion of the trunk takes place without twisting or bending forwards or backwards. When the pelvis starts to move the movement must be stopped. If the quadratus lumborum is shortened, the lumbar spine is kept stiff and the thoracolumbar segments show signs of local compensatory hypermobility. The lower waist crease stays concave.

Possible errors

1. While lying prone the neck is under pressure when the upper trunk is steadied.
2. During the movement there is twisting of the trunk and/or forwards or backwards bending.
3. The pelvis and the legs are not adequately fixed.
4. Palpation of the muscle to be tested is not deep enough and therefore the test is not valid.
5. In the orientation test in the standing position a sideways movement of the pelvis is allowed and also an increased upward movement of the shoulders.

67   Pectoralis major

Tests

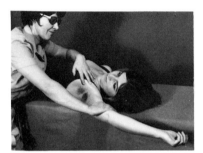

Starting position: Supine lying, with the side to be examined near the edge of the plinth and the arms alongside the body.

Fixation: Before the movement has started there should be a light rotation of the thorax against its expected diagonal direction. The fixation must be applied before elevation of the arm.

Movement: The arm is moved passively from the starting position outwards, across and upwards, so that the palm is directed towards the ceiling.

Normal findings: The upper arm should reach the horizontal plane and with pressure in a vertical and posterior direction it should be possible to increase the range of movement. At the same time the muscle fibres are palpated in the sternal and clavicular parts of the muscle. If there is shortening the upper arm does not reach the horizontal plane and on palpation the tight muscle fibres are detected.

Possible errors

1. The thorax is not adequately fixed before the movement starts and so twisting of the trunk and an increased lumbar lordosis can take place.
2. Instead of fixing the thorax through a diagonal pull there is a vertical push.
3. The pressure during the test is applied not towards the upper but towards the forearm.
4. The direction of the movement is not maintained and so the sternal part of the muscle fibres is not stretched to the necessary extent.

68 The paravertebral back muscles

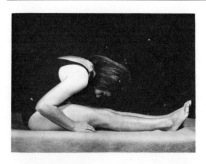

The first phase

Starting position: The patient sits with the legs stretched out on the plinth. The pelvis is as vertical as possible. (If it is tilted backwards this is a sign of shortening of the hamstrings.)
Movement: The patient increases the back flexion to try to touch the forehead on the knees.
Normal findings: The spine must make an even curve. An adult should achieve a distance of 10 cm or less between the forehead and the knees.

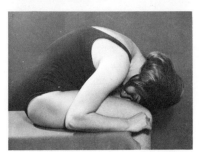

The second phase

Starting position: The patient sits with the knees flexed and the lower legs hanging over the edge of the plinth so that the hamstrings are relaxed.
Movement: Forward bending to the maximum range with the forehead moving towards the knees. The pelvis must not move. If the forward bending of the trunk is distinctly greater than in the first phase it is usually due to increased tilt of the pelvis and shortness of the hamstrings.

Possible errors

1. The test is not performed in two phases.
2. Knee flexion is carried out at the beginning of the movement.
3. The forward bending takes place through tilting the pelvis and not through bending the spine.

69   The trapezius – upper part

Tests

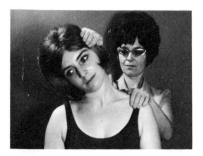

Starting position: Sitting.
Fixation: The shoulder on the side to be tested is fixed from above.
Movement: Passive side flexion of the neck without flexion, extension or rotation.
Normal findings: The range of movement is compared on both sides and the fibres of the trapezius are palpated.

If the patient cannot relax in sitting, the examination can take place supine. The head is moved with the ear to the opposite shoulder while the shoulder on the side to be tested is fixed. The range of movement of both sides must be compared.

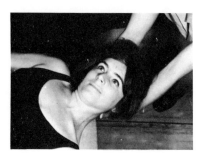

Possible errors

1. The shoulder of the side to be tested is not fixed.
2. The movement takes place with rotation, flexion and extension of the spine.
3. With fixation the skin of the shoulder blade is stretched in the lateral direction (this might be painful).
4. Stretching of the dorsal fibres of the platysma is mistaken for that of the muscle fibres of the trapezius.

70 Levator scapulae

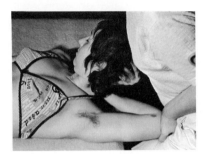

Starting position: Supine lying with the arms alongside the body.
Fixation: The examiner steadies the head with one hand and stabilizes the shoulder with the other.
Movement: Maximal flexion in the cervical spine with rotation and side flexion towards the opposite side. If there is shortening of the levator scapulae, the range of movement is decreased and the muscle insertion on the shoulder blade is painful on palpation.

Possible errors

1. The shoulder is not adequately fixed.
2. The arm of the tested side is not elevated so that the necessary stretch of the fibres of the levator scapulae is not achieved.

Section 3   Examination of hypermobility

Hypermobility is not strictly a disease or a clinical entity and the syndrome is not based exclusively on muscular disorder. However, because it has been assessed in connection with muscle shortening and muscle weakness it should be examined in this context.

There are three principal types of hypermobility, as follows:

1.   Local pathological.
2.   General pathological.
3.   Constitutional.

Local hypermobility can arise in individual movement segments of the spine as a compensatory mechanism for a stiff segment.

A general pathological hypermobility usually arises in disorders of the afferent nerve fibres, for example in tabes dorsalis, some cases of polyneuritis, and similar diseases. It is also seen in disturbances of central muscle tonus regulation such as oligophrenia, and in some cerebellar and extrapyramidal hyperkinetic diseases.

Constitutional hypermobility involves the whole body, although all parts may not be affected to the same extent or even strictly symmetrically. To some degree hypermobility changes with age. The reason is not known, but there is probably a connection with constitutional insufficiency of the mesenchyme or, more generally, "soft tissue weakness". Hypermobility is more common in women. Its estimation is very important not only for pathogenetical analysis in some disorders but also for the total physiotherapy programme. In addition assessment is useful to judge the optimal movement abilities, since hypermobility leads to a decrease in the static weight-bearing tolerance.

An assessment of hypermobility is principally an estimation of the range of movement of the joint. Therefore the measurement of the maximal passive range of movement in the joint is also an assessment of hypermobility. No detailed tests permitting quantitative grading of hypermobility have yet been evolved.

Many different tests exist to show hypermobility. Principally one tries with these tests to assess various parts of the body and to differentiate between the upper and the lower parts. Quite often the hypermobility is found to be more pronounced in the upper or lower part of the body. The differences between the two sides of the body, if present, are slight.

71   Head rotation

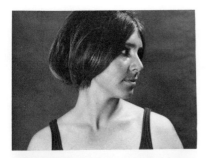

In standing or in sitting the patient turns the head actively first to one side and then to the other. At the end of the range the patient is tested passively in addition to find out if further movement is possible. The normal range is about 80 degrees to each side and the active and the passive movements are almost the same. With hypermobility the head may be rotated actively to over 90 degrees and passively to even more. The symmetry of the rotation each side is compared.

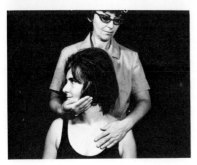

Possible errors

1. Extension and flexion are also allowed.
2. The increased range of movement is not always looked at thoroughly to determine whether the mobility is increased mainly in the cervical cranial part or in the whole cervical spine.

72   High arm cross

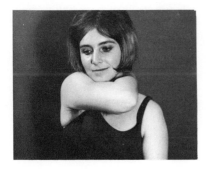

The patient is sitting or standing and puts her arm around the neck from the front towards the opposite side. Normally the elbow almost reaches the median plane of the body and the fingers reach the cervical spine. With hypermobility the range of movement is much greater. The distance the fingers can move across the median plane is measured. The range of movement of the arms must be compared on either side; the subordinate arm may have a slightly larger range of movement.

Possible errors

Errors are not very common.

245

73   Touching the hands behind the back

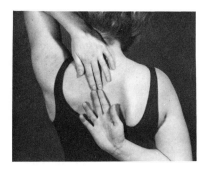

In standing or in sitting the patient tries to bring both hands together behind the back, one from above the shoulder and the other from below. Normally the tips of the fingers can touch without any increase in thoracolumbar lordosis. According to the grade of the hypermobility the patient can put the fingers or the hands on top of each other and in some cases even the wrists. The test is also performed the other way round so that each arm can be compared.

Possible errors

1.   A large increase in lordosis is allowed.
2.   The sides are not compared.

74   Crossing the arms behind the neck

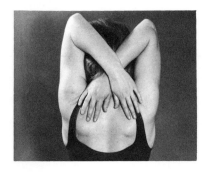

The patient in sitting or lying puts the arms across the neck with the fingers in the direction of the shoulder blades. Normally the tips of the fingers can touch the opposite scapula. With hypermobility the patient can reach part of the shoulder blade or even the whole shoulder blade with the hand or hands.

75   Extension of the elbows

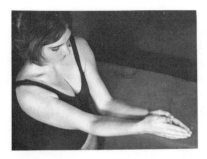

The patient is standing or, even better, sitting. The elbows, lower arms and hands are pressed against each other with the fingers together and maximal flexion in the elbows. The patient tries to extend the elbows without separating them. With a normal range of movement the elbows can be extended to 110 degrees but with hyperextension this angle is much greater.

Possible errors

1.   The elbows are not kept against each other, especially at the end of the range of movement.

76   Movement of the hands:

Test 1

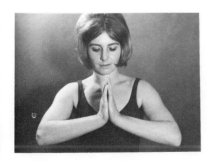

The patient presses the hands against each other in front of the body and overstretches the wrist through a downward movement without parting the hands. Normally it is possible to achieve a 90-degree angle between the hands and the forearms. If this is not possible, it is a sign of shortening of the wrist flexors and the ligaments of the hand. On the other hand, an increase of the hyperextension angle means hypermobility.

Possible errors

The hands are not kept pressed against each other.

77 Movement of the hands:

Test 2

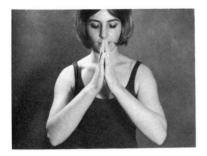

This is in fact the second phase of the previous assessment. The patient pushes the outstretched fingers against each other and the hand is held as a continuation of the forearm. The fingers at the metacarpophalangeal joints are then hyperextended by moving the hands downwards. The hand must stay as a continuation of the forearm throughout the movement. Normally the angle between the palms is 80 degrees. With hypermobility this angle is much greater.

Possible errors

1. The exact position of the hands in the axis of the forearm is not checked.
2. The outstretched fingers are not pressed against each other along their whole surface.

78 Forward flexion of the back

Tests

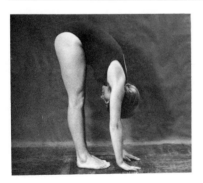

The patient is in standing and bends forwards with straight legs and the feet together as in the Thomayer (Néri) test. The bending of the back as a whole and the tilting of the pelvis and the curve of the spine are observed. If there is a difference of hypermobility in the upper and lower halves of the body, especially when this is due to shortened hamstrings, the pelvis is tilted just a little. When there is shortening of the paravertebral lumbar muscles, there is a compensatory increase of kyphosis in the thoracic spine and the lumbar spine remains more or less straight. Normally the patient can touch the floor with the fingertips. The hypermobility is graded depending on how much of the hand touches the floor, for instance the fingertips, the fingers or the whole hand.

Possible errors

1. Flexion in the knee joint and forward bending are not observed properly.
2. The kyphosis and the tilting of the pelvis are not differentiated.

79 Side flexion of the back

Tests

The patient is in standing with the feet together and bends sideways, at the same time moving the hand downwards against the outside of the thigh. The shoulder must not be lifted in compensation and the pelvis must not be moved sideways. Normally a plumb line dropped from the shoulder crease should come to the intergluteal line.

With hypermobility the side flexion is increased and so the plumb line hangs from the shoulder crease towards the contralateral side. In the case of shortening, particularly of the quadratus lumborum (see p. 239) the plumb line does not reach the intergluteal line.

One may also register how far down below the knee joint the patient can reach. This test is not very accurate because it also depends on the length of the arms.

Possible errors

1. Rotation towards the backward movement of the trunk is allowed.
2. There is a shift forward or a backward movement of the pelvis.

80 Sitting down between the heels

Tests

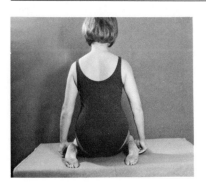

The patient is kneeling and attempts to sit down between the heels. Normally the bottom reaches a line between the heels. With hypermobility the patient can sit down on the floor. With shortening, especially of the rectus femoris, the bottom stays above the heels.

Possible errors

Faults are not very common but the trunk must not be bent forwards.

81 Forward bending in kneeling

Tests

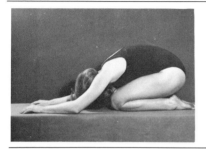

The patient sits on her heels and tries to place the trunk on her thighs. Normally this is possible. With hypermobility it is very easy and the patient can put her trunk between the knees almost down on the floor.

Possible errors

1. The bottom is not pressed down on the heels during the full movement.

82 Side flexion in kneeling

Tests

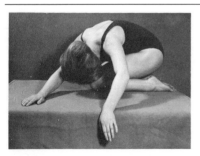

The patient sits on the heels with the toes directed backwards and simultaneously performs maximal forward and sideways bending. The evenness of the movement is observed together with the range of the movement.

Possible errors

The test is not very objective.

83 A summary of assessment

During examination it would be very uncomfortable and difficult for the patient to continuously turn around, stand up, sit down and so on, which is necessary if each test is performed from grade 1 to grade 5. The following tables list the tests in the order in which the patient should be assessed. The assessment is therefore first carried out in one position and then in another.

Tests

In standing:
Pelvis: elevation grade 3
Hip joint: rotation grade 2a
Ankle joint: plantar flexion grades 3, 4, 5

In sitting:
Trunk: rotation grade 2a
Shoulder blade: abduction grades 0, 1, 2, 4, 5
                  adduction grades 0, 1, 2
                  elevation grades 3, 4, 5
Shoulder joint: flexion under 90 degrees grades 3, 4, 5
                abduction grades 3, 4, 5
                extension in abduction grades 0, 1, 2
                flexion from abduction grades 0, 1, 2
Elbow joint: flexion grades 2b, 3, 4, 5
            extension grade 2b
Lower arms: supination grades 3, 4, 5
           pronation grades 3, 4, 5
Wrist joint: flexion all grades
         extension all grades
Fingers: all tests, all grades
Hip joint: flexion grades 3, 4, 5
Ankle joint: tibialis anterior grades 3, 4, 5
Toe joints: All tests all grades

In side lying:
Neck: flexion grade 2
      extension grade 2
Trunk: extension grade 2

In side lying (on the side not to be tested):
Shoulder joint: extension grade 2
               flexion to 90 degrees grade 2
Hip joint: abduction grades 3, 4
Ankle joint: peronei grades 3, 4, 5

In side lying (on the side of the leg to be tested):
Hip joint: flexion grade 2
        extension grade 2
        abduction grades 3, 4, 5
Knee joint: extension grade 2
          flexion grade 2

Ankle joint: tibialis anterior grade 2
          tibialis posterior grades 3, 4, 5
          plantar flexion grades 0, 1, 2

In prone lying:
Neck: extension grades 0, 1, 3, 4, 5
Trunk: extension grades 0, 1, 3, 4, 5
Shoulder blades: adduction grades 3, 4, 5
                 innervation grades, 0, 1, 2
                 caudal movement all grades
Shoulder joint: extension grades 0, 1, 3, 4, 5
                extension in abduction grades 3, 4, 5
                rotation all grades
Elbow joint: extension grades 3, 4, 5
Lower arms: supination grades 0, 1, 3
           pronation grade 2
Hip joint: extension grades 0, 1, 3, 4, 5
Knee joint: flexion grades 0, 1, 3, 4, 5
Ankle joint: plantar flexion grades 3, 4, 5

In supine lying:
Neck: flexion grades 0, 1, 3, 4, 5
Trunk: flexion all grades
      rotation grades 0, 1, 2b, 3, 4, 5
Shoulder blade: serratus anterior grade 3
Shoulder joint: flexion to 90 degrees grades 0, 1
                abduction to 90 degrees grades 0, 1, 2
                flexion from abduction grades 3, 4, 5
Elbow joint: flexion grades 0, 1, 2a
            extension grades 0, 1, 2a
Lower arm: pronation grades 0, 1
Pelvis: elevation grades 0, 1, 2, 4, 5
Hip joint: flexion grades 0, 1
        abduction grades 0, 1, 2
        adduction grades 0, 1, 2
        rotation grades 0, 1, 2b, 3, 4, 5
Knee joint: extension grades 0, 1, 3, 4, 5
Ankle joint: tibialis posterior grades 0, 1, 2
          tibialis anterior grades 0, 1
          peronei grades 0, 1, 2
Toe joints: all tests all grades

Appendix:

Examples of schemes for muscle tests

Muscle test

Hospital:　　　　　　　　　　Born:　　　　　　　Address:

Name:　　　　　　　　　　　　　　　　　　　　　Diagnosis:

Right						Face								Left
	/ 19	/ 19	/ 19	/ 19	/ 19	Movement	Muscle	Innervation	/ 19	/ 19	/ 19	/ 19	/ 19	
Face						Right eyebrow, crosses forehead	Frontalis	N. VII, facialis						Face
						Close the eyelid	Orbicularis oculi	''						
						Draw together the eyebrows	Corrugator supercilii	''						
						Trace a line between the eyebrows	Procerus	''						
						Press the nostrils medial position	Nasalis	''						
						Close the mouth, purse the lips	Orbicularis oris	''						
						Draw the mouth up and sideways causing dimple formation	Zygomaticus major Risorius	''						
Face						Draw the top lip sideways, part the lips upwards and sideways	Levator anguli oris	''						Face
						Draw the lower lip down and sideways	Depressor anguli oris Depressor labii inf.	''						
						Press the lower lip up and hollow the cheeks	Mentalis	''						
						Stretch the skin on the cheeks and neck	Platysma	''						
						Stretch the inner part of the chin	Buccinator	''						
						Draw the jaw up	Masseter	N. V., trigeminus						

Right					Face			Left					
/ 19	/ 19	/ 19	/ 19	/ 19	Movement	Muscle	Innervation	/ 19	/ 19	/ 19	/ 19	/ 19	
					Draw the jaw up and back	Temporalis	,,						
					Draw the jaw forwards and upwards	Pterygoidei	,,						
Sign					Code text for the following sides. NB:Does not count for face muscles. 5: Full movement against strong resistance 4: Full movement against less resistance 3: Full movement against gravity 2: Full movement without gravity 1: Without movement 0: No contraction S = spasm; SS = severe spasm; C = contracture; CC = severe contracture; RM = reduced mobility; F = shortening; FF = severe shortening								Sign

Muscle test

Hospital: Born: Address:
Name: Diagnosis:

Right									Left			
/ 19	/ 19	/ 19	/ 19	Movement		Muscle		Peripheral innervation	Segmental innervation	/ 19	/ 19	/ 19	/ 19
					dig. II		I	Medianus	C8–T1				
				Flexion MCP	dig. III	Lumbricalis	II	Medianus	C8–T1				
					dig. IV		III	Ulnaris	C8–T1				
					dig. V		IV	Ulnaris	C8–T1				
				Extension MCP	dig. II			Radialis	C6–C8				
					dig. III	Extensor digitorum		Radialis	C6–C8				
					dig. IV			Radialis	C6–C8				
					dig. V			Radialis	C6–C8				
				Adduction MCP	dig. II	Interosseus palmaris	I	Ulnaris	C8–T1				
					dig. IV		II	Ulnaris	C8–T1				
					dig. V		III	Ulnaris	C8–T1				
				Abduction MCP	dig. II	Interosseus dorsalis	I	Ulnaris	C8–T1				
					dig. III		II	Ulnaris	C8–T1				
					dig. III		III	Ulnaris	C8–T1				
					dig. IV		IV	Ulnaris	C8–T1				
					dig. V	Abductor digiti min.		Ulnaris	C8–T1				
					dig. II			Medianus	C7–T1				
				Flexion PIP	dig. III	Flexor digit. superficialis		Medianus	C7–T1				
					dig. IV			Medianus	C7–T1				
					dig. V			Medianus	C7–T1				

Finger with 3 phalanges

254

Right									Left				
	/ 19	/ 19	/ 19	/ 19	Movement		Muscle	Peripheral innervation	Segmental innervation	/ 19	/ 19	/ 19	/ 19
Finger with 3 phalanges					Flexion DIP	dig. II	Flexor digit. profundus	Medianus	C7–T1					**Finger with 3 phalanges**
						dig. III		Ulnaris (Medianus)	C7–T1					
						dig. IV		Ulnaris	C7–T1					
						dig. V		Ulnaris	C7–T1					
					Opposition	dig. V	Opponens dig. minimi	Ulnaris	C7–T1					
Thumb					Opposition	dig. I	Opponens pollicis	Medianus	C6–C7					**Thumb**
					Adduction	with hand held flat	Adductor pollicis Flexor pollicis brevis	Ulnaris Medianus + Ulnaris	C6–C7					
						hand joint flap	Interosseus dors. I	Ulnaris	C8–T1					
					Abduction	with hand held flat	Abductor poll. longus Extensor poll. brevis	Radialis	C6–C7					
						hand joints flap	Abductor poll. brevis Flexor poll. brevis	Medianus Medianus + Ulnaris	C6–C7					
					Flexion MCP I		Flexor poll. brevis, caput superficiale Flexor poll. brevis caput profundum	Medianus Radialis	C6–C7					
					Extension MCP 1		Extensor poll. brevis	Radialis	C6–C7					
					Flexion IP		Flexor poll. longus	Medianus	C7–C8					
					Extension IP		Extensor poll. longus	Radialis	C6–C8					
Sign					Remarks									**Sign**

Muscle test

Hospital: Born: Address:

Name: Diagnosis:

				Right Movement	Muscle	Peripheral innervation	Segmental innervation					
	/ 19	/ 19	/ 19	/ 19	Movement	Muscle	Peripheral innervation	Segmental innervation	/ 19	/ 19	/ 19	/ 19	
Neck					Flexion bending forward	Scaleni, long. coll+cap.	Plexus cervicalis	C1–C6					Neck
					Flexion shortening forward	Sternocleido-mastoideus	Accessorius Plexus cervicalis	N.XI C2–C3					
					Extension	Trapezius, pars. sup.	Accessorius Plexus cervicalis	N.XI C2–C3					
Trunk					Flexion	Rectus abdominis	Intercostales 6–12	T6–T12					Trunk
						Transversus abdominis	Intercostales 7–12 iliohypogastricus	T7–T12 L1					
					Extension (thor.) (lumb).	Erector spinae Quadratus lumborum	Rr. dorsales, subcost., plexus lumb.	L2–C2 T12–L1–4					
					Rotation	sin. obliq. ext. abd. dx., dx. obliq. int. abd. sin.	Intercostales 5–12 8–12	T5–T12 T8–T12					
Back					Elevation	Quadratus lumborum	Subcostalis Plexus lumbalis	T12 L1–L4					Back
Hip joint					Flexion	Iliopsoas	Plexus lumbalis Femoralis	L1–L4					Hip joint
					Extension	Gluteus maximus Biceps, semitend., semimembr.	Gluteus inf. Tibialis, fibularis	L5–S2 L4–S1					
					Extension	Gluteus maximus	Gluteus inf.	L5–S2					
					Adduction	Adductores	Obturatorius	L2–L4					
					Abduction	Gluteus medius	Gluteus sup.	L4–S1					
					Lateral rotation	Obturatorius ext. Obt. int., quadratus, gemelli	Obturatorius Plexus sacralis	L3–L4 L4–S2					
					Medial rotation	Gluteus minimus tensor fasc. latae	Gluteus sup.	L4–S1					
					Flexion	Biceps femoris c. long. c. brev.	Ischiadicus	L4–S1					

256

Right													Left
	/ 19	/ 19	/ 19	/ 19	Movement	Muscle	Peripheral innervation	Sègmental innervation	/ 19	/ 19	/ 19	/ 19	
Knee joint					Flexion	Semimembranosus Semitendinosus	Ischiadicus	L1–S1					Knee joint
					Extension	Rectus femoris	Femoralis	L2–L4					
					Extension	Vasti med., lat., intermedius	Femoralis	L2–L4					
Ankle					Plantar flexion	Triceps surae	Ischiadicus – tib.	L4–S1					Ankle
					Plantar flexion	Soleus	Ischiadicus – tib.	L4–S1					
					Supination and dorsal flexion	Tibialis ant.	Ischiadicus – per. prof.	L4–L5					
					Supination with plantar flexion	Tibialis post.	Ischiadicus – tib.	L4–S1					
					Pronation (plantar)	Peroneus longus och brevis	Ischiadicus – per. sup.	L4–S1					
Toe					Flexion MTP-led	Lumbricales I, II, III, IV	Tibialis - plant med. - plant. lat.	L5–S1 S1–S2					Toe
					Flexion MTP-led I	Flexor hall. brevis	Tibialis-plant. med. och. lat.	L5–S1 S1–S2					
					Extension MTP-led	Extensor dig. long. och. brev., ext. hall. brev.	Ischiadicus – per. prof.	L4–S1					
					Flexion PIP-led	Flexor dig. brevis	Tibialis – plant. med.	L5–S1					
					Flexion DIP-led	Flexor dig. longus	Ischiadicus – tib.	L5–S2					
					Flexion IP-led I	Flexor hall. longus	Ischiadicus – tib.	L5–S2					
					Extensor IP-led I	Extensor hall. longus	Ischiadicus – per. prof.	L4–S1					
					Adduction	Interossei plant. Adductor hall.	Tibialis – plant. lat.	S1–S2					
					Abduction	Interos. dors., abd. dig. min. Abductor hall.	Tibialis – plant. lat. Tibialis – plant. med.	S1–S2 L5–S1					
Sign					Remarks:								Sign

Hospital: Born: Address:

Name: Diagnosis:

					Movement	Muscle	Peripheral innervation	Segmental innervation					
Right													Left
	/ 19	/ 19	/ 19	/ 19					/ 19	/ 19	/ 19	/ 19	
Shoulder blade					Adduction	Trapezius, pars. med. rhomboidei major, minor	Accessorius, plexus cervic. dorsalis scap.	N. XI C2–C4					Shoulder blade
					Adduction and caudal shortening	Trapezius, pars. inf.	Accessorius Plexus cervic	N. XI C2–C4					
					Elevation	Trapezius, pars. sup. Levator scapulae	Access. och plex. cervic. Dorsalis scapulae	N. XI C2–C5					
					Abduction and rotation	Serratus ant.	Thoracicus longus	C5–C7					
Shoulder joint					Flexion	Deltoideus. pars. clavic. Coracobrachialis	Axillaris Musculocutaneus	C5–C6 C5–C7					Shoulder joint
					Extension	Latis. dorsi, teres, major, deltoideus, pars. scapul.	Thoracodorsalis, subscapularis axillaris	C5–C8					
					Abduction	Deltoideus, pars. acrom. Supraspinatus	Axillaris Suprascapularis	C5–C6 C4–C5					
					Extension with abduction	Deltoideus, pars. scapul.	Axillaris	C5–C6					
					Flexion with abduction	Pectoralis major	Thoracici	C5–T1					
					Lateral rotation	Infraspinatus Teres minor	Suprascapularis Axillaris	C4–C5 C5–C6					
					Medial rotation	Subscap., teres maj., pectoralis major, latissimus dorsi	Subscapul. thoracici thoracodors.	C5–T1					
Elbow joint					Flexion with supination of the forearm	Biceps brachii	Musculocutaneus	C5–C6					Elbow joint
					Flexion with pronation of the forearm	Brachialis	Musculocutaneus	C5–C6					
					Flexion with forearm in midposition	Brachioradialis	Radialis	C5–C6					

				Movement	Muscle	Peripheral innervation	Segmental innervation					
	/19	/19	/19	/19					/19	/19	/19	/19
Forearm					Extension	Triceps brachii Anconeus	Radialis	C6–C8					**Forearm**
					Supination	Biceps brachii Supinator	Musculocutaneus Radialis	C5–C6					
					Pronation	Pronator teres Pronator quadratus	Medianus	C6–C7 C7–T1					
Wrist					Flexion and ulnar flexion	Flexor carpi ulnaris	Ulnaris	C7–T1					**Wrist**
					Flexion and radial flexion	Flexor carpi radialis	Medianus	C6–C8					
					Extension and ulnar flexion	Extensor carpi ulnaris	Radialis	C6–C8					
					Extension and radial flexion	Extensor carpi rad. long. och brev.	Radialis	C6–C8					
Finger with 3 phalanges					Flexion MCP-led	Lumbric. I o. II, III, IV, och interossei palm. dors.	Medianus Ulnaris	C6–C7 C8–T1					**Finger with 3 phalanges**
					Extension MCP-led	Extensor dig., ind., dig. min.	Radialis	C6–C8					
					Adduction MCP-led	Interossei palm.	Ulnaris	C8–T1					
					Abduction MCP-led	Interossei dors.	Ulnaris	C8–T1					
					Flexion PIP-led	Abd. dig. min. Flexor dig. superf.	Medianus	C7–T1					
					Flexion DIP-led	Flexor dig. prof. for 2 For 3–5 finger	Medianus Ulnaris	C7–T1					
					Opposition of dig. V	Opponens dig. min.	Ulnaris	C8–T1					
Thumb					Opposition of thumb	Opponens pollicis	Medianus	C6–C7					**Thumb**
					Adduction CMC-led I	Adductor pollicis	Ulnaris	C8–T1					

259

	/ 19	/ 19	/ 19	/ 19	Movement	Muscle	Peripheral innervation	Segmental innervation	/ 19	/ 19	/ 19	/ 19	
Thumb					Abduction CMC-led I	Abductor pollicis longus Abductor pollicis brevis	Radialis Medianus	C6–C7					**Thumb**
					Flexion MCP-led I	Flexor poll. brev. c. superf. c. prof.	Medianus Ulnaris	C6–C7					
					Extension MCP-led	Extensor poll. brevis	Radialis	C6–C7					
					Flexion IP-led I	Flexor poll. longus	Medianus	C7–C8					
					Extension IP-led I	Extensor poll. longus	Radialis	C6–C8					
Sign					Remarks:								**Sign**